Health promotion

This is the first book as such in the field of health promotion that attempts to trace the disciplinary roots of the subject. With many practical examples of applied theory, it relates the theoretical with the practical to form an essential reference for academics and practitioners alike.

In terms of theoretical development, health promotion is at a crossroads. Over the last twenty years or so, it has emerged from its roots in public health and health education to become a central force in the 'new' public health movement. This has been accompanied by a proliferation in papers concerned with research, theory, and the discipline of health promotion, such that it now demands to be recognized as an emerging and discrete discipline.

This book debates whether it has yet reached a stage of independence from its disciplinary roots or if it is, in fact, still a product of a multi-disciplinary base. Contributions from experts in the fields of psychology, sociology, education, and epidemiology, the primary feeder disciplines, explain how concepts and theories from these academic fields have helped to shape health promotion theory, whilst contributors from the secondary feeder disciplines of economics, philosophy, social policy, communications, and social marketing argue that their disciplines offer further conceptual bases for the academic development of health promotion.

Robin Bunton is Senior Lecturer in Social Policy at the University of Teesside. **Gordon Macdonald** is Head of Professional Development at the Health Promotion Authority for Wales. Both lecture at the Institute of Health Promotion, University of Wales College of Medicine, in Cardiff.

Health promotion

Disciplines and diversity

Edited by
Robin Bunton
and
Gordon Macdonald

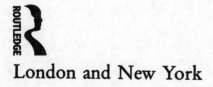

London and New York

First published 1992
by Routledge
11 New Fetter Lane, London EC4P 4EE

Simultaneously published in the USA and Canada
by Routledge
29 West 35th Street, New York, NY 10001

Reprinted 1993 (twice) and 1995

Typeset in Garamond by
Falcon Typographic Art Ltd, Edinburgh
Printed and bound in Great Britain by
Mackays of Chatham PLC, Chatham, Kent

British Library Cataloguing in Publication Data
A catalogue record for this book is available from the British Library

Library of Congress Cataloguing in Publication Data
A catalogue record for this book is available from the Library of Congress

ISBN 0-415-07555-6 (hbk)
ISBN 0-415-05981-X (pbk)

Contents

Contributors

Paul Bennett

Paul Bennett is a lecturer in Health Psychology at the University of Wales College of Cardiff. Until recently he was a Senior Research Officer with the Health Promotion Authority for Wales. He is a founder member of both the British Psychological Society's Section of Health Psychology and the European Health Psychology Society. His present research interests include cardiovascular health psychology and the relationships between psychological variables and health-related behaviours.

Robin Bunton

Robin Bunton is Director of Alcohol Concern Wales/Gweithgor Alcohol Cymru and Lecturer at the Institute for Health Promotion, University of Wales College of Medicine, Cardiff. His current research interests include sociology of public health, substance misuse policy, and mental health.

David Cohen

David Cohen is a Principal Lecturer in Health Economics at the Polytechnic of Wales. He previously spent five years as a Research Fellow at the Health Economics Research Unit at Aberdeen University. His main area of research interest is the economics of prevention and he has co-authored a book on this subject.

Ray Hodgson

Ray Hodgson is Head of the Department of Psychology for South Glamorgan Health Authority (and Honorary Professor of the University of Wales). He was a member of the Health Promotion Authority for Wales from its inception until 1991. His area of specialism is alcohol- and drug-related psychological disorders and he is a World Health Organization

Adviser in this field. He is on the Editorial Board of the *British Journal of Addiction* and the *Journal of Mental Health*.

Craig Lefebvre

Craig Lefebvre received his PhD in Clinical Psychology from North Texas State University, and has held post-doctoral fellowships in behavioural medicine at the University of Virginia Medical Centre and in cardiovascular behavioural medicine research at the University of Pittsburgh. He is an Associate Professor (Research) in the Department of Community Health, Brown University, and has been the Intervention Director of the Pawtucket Heart Health Program since 1984. He has written and lectured widely on social marketing approaches to public health interventions.

Gordon Macdonald

Gordon Macdonald was previously head of a health promotion service in Cambridgeshire in England but is now Head of Professional Development at the Health Promotion Authority for Wales in Cardiff and also Course Director on the MSc in Health Promotion and Health Education at the Institute for Health Promotion in the University of Wales College of Medicine. He has undertaken a number of consultancies for the World Health Organization and currently co-ordinates the WHO-sponsored International Summer School held annually in Cardiff in the UK and is also Associate Editor for the academic journal *Health Promotion International*. His current research interests include curriculum development in professional education and health education curriculum innovation in secondary schools.

Don Rawson

Don Rawson is a Principal Lecturer in Health Education Research at the Southbank Polytechnic, London. His interest in health promotion emerged from his researching the social psychology of decision making. He is currently studying the social representation of health actions.

Andrew Tannahill

Andrew Tannahill trained in community medicine (now public health medicine) in the East of Scotland before setting up a department of health promotion at East Anglian Regional Health Authority. His contribution to this book was made while he was Senior Lecturer in Public Health Medicine at the University of Glasgow with teaching responsibilities in both epidemiology and health promotion. He has since been appointed General Manager of the Health Education Board for Scotland. The views expressed in his chapter are entirely personal, and should not be attributed in any way to the Health Education Board for Scotland.

Nicki Thorogood

Nicki Thorogood teaches sociology of health at Middlesex Polytechnic and the Royal Free School of Medicine and is Development Officer for the City and Hackney Health Authority Young People's Project. Her current research interests include sociology of public health, sexuality, race, and gender.

Katherine Weare

Katherine Weare is a lecturer in health education in the Faculty of Education and visiting lecturer in primary medical care in the Faculty of Medicine at the University of Southampton. Her responsibilities include being Director of the Health Education Unit, Co-ordinator of Initial Teacher Education, and Tutor on the MA in Health Education. Her current interests include developing health education in training of doctors and teachers, and setting up in-service courses for those involved in health education in Britain and in Europe.

Foreword
Vital signs of health promotion

Health promotion has emerged in the last decade as an important force to improve both the quality and quantity of people's lives. Sometimes termed 'the new public health' it seeks to support and encourage a participative social movement that enables individuals and communities to take control over their own health. Whilst discussions have focused usefully on the 'added value' of health promotion compared to other health development approaches, little attention has been given to the nature and content of health promotion as an academic discipline, or more accurately an alliance of academic disciplines.

The overall quest for health promotion is to raise the level of health populations in the most effective, ethical, and equitable way possible. This requires a firm understanding of the contributions that a range of 'feeder' disciplines can offer. These are as diverse as epidemiology, education, sociology, communications, psychology, marketing, social policy, philosophy, and economics. This inter-disciplinary academic base to health promotion could be mirrored by common features of use to practitioners thereby relating theory to practice. These common features or 'vital signs' may provide an indication that health promotion is alive and well.

Drawing on our academic and service experience in Wales we think that there is a common set of factors which indicates that health promotion is capable of dynamic development. These vital signs might include the following ten factors:

Understanding and responding to people's needs, to enable people to take control over their health or empower them through a people-centred approach, explicitly demonstrated.

Building on sound theoretical principles and understanding by firmly rooting health promotion in the relevant arts and sciences (outlined in this book). Practitioners should be able to justify their actions on a theoretical basis since nothing is as practical as a good theory.

Demonstrating a sense of direction and coherence by developing a logical strategy with an overarching vision or 'strategic intent' from which practical programmes of action may be devised and monitored.

Collecting, analysing, and using information through comprehensive needs assessments and programme evaluations. A good information management system allows for the conversion of data into intelligence. Information itself can also be a powerful intervention and there should be active links with the media.

Reorienting key decision makers – a major target group for the enabling, mediating, and advocating roles of health promotion are those individuals who control policies and resources. Health promoters need to show that they are actively working 'upstream'.

Connecting with all sectors and settings that impact on life is essential if health promotion is to be fully effective. There should be demonstrable outreach programmes responsive to the opportunities available.

Using complementary approaches at both individual and environmental levels supports that previous factor and allows for a mutually interactive and supportive programme of action at both the individual and environmental level. If this is not addressed there is a danger of 'victim blaming' on the one hand or social engineering on the other.

Encouraging participation and ownership through a people-centred approach creates that opportunity for a more effective delivery of health promotion programmes.

Providing technical and managerial training and support is fundamental if the full potential of a large number of change agents within the population is to be realized.

Undertaking specific actions and programmes, the real focus for health promotion, is critical if analysis paralysis is to be avoided. Examples should be evident from a combination of intervention approaches including personal education and development, mass media information and education, personal services, community action, organizational development, environmental measures, and economic and regulatory activities.

If these 'vital signs' of health promotion are to be fully maintained, those working in the field will need to have a firm grasp of the essential skills and understanding which are drawn from a range of disciplines across the arts and sciences.

This is why *Health Promotion* provides a most valuable and timely addition to the literature for both students and practitioners. As well as describing the principle theories and issues relevant for health promotion, the editors have pulled together contributions that make the vital link between theory and practice, so important in a field such as health promotion. Examples are given of health promotion programmes that have made use of the theoretical principles from these disciplines.

This book, as well as being a sound academic reader, is also an important self-help aid – thereby ensuring health promotion remains healthy.

John Catford
Professor of Health Promotion
University of Wales College of Medicine

Acknowledgements

We would like to thank a number of people who helped at various stages in the production of this volume: Lesley Jones, Sally Baldwin, and Simon Murphy for reading through some early draft chapters, Jenny Saunders for helping to compile the glossary to the text.

Special thanks to Jane Bennett and Eiluned Williams for their diligence and patience in typing much of the text. Finally, thanks to Elisabeth Tribe for her support in production and editing.

Introduction

Robin Bunton and Gordon Macdonald

'Health Promotion' is rapidly establishing itself as an important force within the 'New Public Health', itself an important feature of contemporary approaches to health and health care provision. Whilst debates have raged around definitions of health promotion and the differences between health promotion and health education, there has been little concern for the nature of the knowledge base being drawn upon by health promoters and researchers discussing such topics. This neglect is curious considering the wealth of new conceptual development emerging in and around the health promotion field.

The stock of health promotion texts and journals is growing rapidly as is the number of courses at undergraduate and postgraduate levels. Health promotion is increasingly entering the discourse of a wide range of professional journals. With such evident and unprecedented growth in the knowledge base informing health promotion there is a need to assess and keep a perspective on the variety of contributions being made to the field of study. Health promotion is a multi-disciplinary endeavour. Different forms of expertise inform practice and research and are drawn upon to suit different purposes at different times, often with little conception of the appropriateness of overall disciplinary balance. This volume is an attempt to inject some critical awareness into the use of theory in health promotion research and practice. The contributions have been written to draw attention to the forms of knowledge currently contributing to health promotion. They illustrate their range and depth and give examples of how such theory either is being or could be drawn upon to promote health.

The academic roots of health promotion lie in what might be called the primary feeder disciplines, that is, psychology, education, epidemiology, and sociology. More recently, secondary feeder disciplines such as social policy, communications theory, marketing, economics, and philosophy have also made substantial contributions. Underlying previous development in health education and to a large extent evident in health promotion also are the medical disciplines. A medical contribution has often been and still is present in the form of an underlying influence but, with the exception of epidemiology, has been excluded from this collection for a number of reasons. In the first place it was felt that a medical perspective is acknowledged in many of the contributions. Second, the object and focus of much of health promotion work rests, certainly at practice level, on a medical perspective, though more often from a social medicine viewpoint. Third, the place of medicine within health promotion has been problematic. Indeed much of health promotion literature has developed in reaction to a traditional medical perspective on health. The 'bio-medical model' has been found restrictive for the purposes of health promotion.

A central theme of health promotion is to develop interventions that do not resort to institutionalized medical forms of care. As such it fits in with more general moves away from state welfare provision and within a new public policy environment. It is possible to consider health promotion as a frontier of contemporary policy and cultural change (Beattie 1991). Health promotion is now a growing part of industrialized health care systems, and is increasingly an integral part of primary care provision. It is representative of fundamental shifts in the relationship between the state and citizens.

Central to health promotion is a commitment to multi-sectoral action. To be successful, collaboration in practice must be matched by collaboration in theory. This can be done only by taking multi-disciplinarity seriously, acknowledging the potential and the pitfalls of such an enterprise. A step in this direction is to bring together contributions to health promotion as a discipline(s) in one volume. Along with other work this exercise can contribute to a much needed self-consciousness about the place of theory (and competing theory) in health promotion (McQueen 1991). Ultimately the success of this kind of self-examination will be dependent upon how it facilitates future development and progress, which may suggest other goals for the year 2000 and beyond.

The book's approach then is designed to lay out relevant theories from both primary and secondary feeder disciplines and to relate these theories to health promotion conception, planning, and practice. In some cases, as in Chapter 2 on the contribution of psychology, the disciplinary contribution is perhaps more readily apparent than in others. Nevertheless, we believe that all the chapters in this book reflect the central role these nine disciplines have played in the development of health promotion thinking and practice. We cannot claim that these chapters constitute an exhaustive list of all relevant disciplines, but we believe they form a substantial part of the principal body of knowledge currently informing health promotion. The book is designed to lay out some of the sources and types of theory that can be drawn upon by health promotion practitioners. We are aware that current theory has largely been the product of the efforts of practitioners as a result of reflection on their own practice. This will no doubt continue to be an important source of theoretical development in an essentially practice-centred field.

Although there is no obvious or 'natural' division to be made amongst the contributing disciplines, we have deliberately put the four 'primary feeder disciplines' at the beginning of this collection and concentrated on the 'secondary feeder disciplines' in Chapters 6 to 10 in the second part of the book. We are aware that this division is to some extent arbitrary and that contributing authors and others might prefer an alternative order. Our ordering principle is based upon what we consider the most significant contributions of each discipline to health promotion to date. We fully expect this order to be contested and changed in the coming decades.

Our opening chapter is intended to put health promotion in a public health context and examine its relationship with health education. This is done by tracing the development of health promotion over the last three decades and arguing that it is intimately linked to the conceptual development of the new public health, with its own relatively autonomous trajectory building upon the conceptual ideas of health education. The main argument of the first chapter, however, is that health promotion is currently undergoing a change characteristic of paradigm shifts in disciplinary or scientific knowledge development. This argument is not uncontestable and is challenged by *Rawson* in Chapter 10 where he argues that there is insufficient evidence of a paradigm shift and that such claims are illusory. *Rawson* is more interested in how health and health promotion relate to fundamental philosophical notions to do with scientific method, epistemology, and the search for truth, and how consideration of these can help to shape and determine future health education and health promotion models and theories.

In the second chapter, *Bennett and Hodgson* examine the contribution psychology, and in particular social psychology, has made to the development of health promotion theory and practice. They argue that psychological theories, especially social learning theory, attribution theory, and the theory of reasoned action, contribute, through the health belief model, to an under-standing of an explanation for human behaviour essential to health. They apply these theories to case studies in health promotion including sexual behaviour change in an HIV programme, promoting sensible drinking, and reducing coronary heart disease risk behaviour. Finally, there is a brief commentary on the contribution of communication theory in the development of major intervention programmes. Communication theory, and in particular innovation-diffusion theory, is further analysed by *Macdonald* in the penultimate chapter. Classical innovation-diffusion theory is described with some illustrative health promotion examples but the author does devote some space to criticizing weak links in the innovation-diffusion chain. Specific areas for concern, he argues, are problems to do with research design and the effects of innovation-diffusion on equity, particularly in a developing world context.

Thorogood's chapter on the relevance of sociology to health promotion begins by providing a synopsis of what the discipline of sociology is about. The author claims that, if sociology is concerned with providing an understanding of how society is organized and analysing the social processess within it, then it has a lot to offer health promotion. After commenting on medical conceptions of health and illness, the author examines social variables that can affect health, such as class, gender, age, and culture. Chapter 3 provides a number of useful examples of health promotion programmes that have not drawn upon sociological method and finishes by asking whether health promotion acts as an agent of social regulation. This theme is picked up in Chapter 7 by *Bunton* who begins with an introduction to the concept of healthy public policy, arguing that there is a convergence of interests between health promoters and social policy in this area. The principal theme in the chapter is that a concern for healthy public policy takes health promotion firmly into the social policy arena and that health promotion can and does benefit from the study of the social policy process. Examples of the application of such analysis are given with particular reference to the promotion of healthy public policy on substance misuse. Different perspectives on the policy process are emphasized.

The third primary feeder discipline covered in the book is education and *Weare*'s chapter gives many useful examples of health education materials, used in both formal and informal education settings, that have borrowed from education theory and methodology. The author concentrates on notions of autonomy before moving on to examine effective ways to educate, emphasizing the need to recognize and employ a growth and development perspective. This should give equal importance to cognitive, emotional, and social dimensions in an educational strategy.

Tannahill proposes a more radical contribution, from epidemiology, to the disciplinary development of health promotion. The first half of the chapter provides the reader with an overview of epidemiology, essentially study of the distribution and determinants of disease, whilst the second half is centred around a critical analysis of the shortcomings of convential understandings of epidemiology. The author calls for a new approach that roots the epidemiology of health (as opposed to disease) firmly in the health promotion camp.

The second part of the book, which concentrates on secondary feeder disciplines, starts with an examination of the contribution economics can make to the study of health promotion. *Cohen* argues that economics can provide a framework for considering how efficiently health promotion achieves its objectives and for the most cost-effective use of resources. In particular, through a description of cost-benefit, cost-efficiency, and cost-unit analyses, the author applies economic theory to a practical health promotion example, namely a reduction in smoking prevalence rates. By using broad objectives economics can, the author argues, introduce informed choice in deciding which programme option to adopt.

Chapter 8 by *Lefebvre* considers the contribution of social marketing to health promotion. This chapter complements other chapters in the book, particularly Chapter 9, since social marketing is concerned with the introduction and dissemination of new ideas or issues within a community. Describing eight characteristics of social marketing the author is emphatic that social marketing is not about social control but is a new problem-solving approach aimed at tackling ill health and social problems. Through careful planning and implementation, the author argues, it can be an effective strategy for social change.

The volume ends with the contribution of philosophy to health promotion. *Rawson*'s chapter is perhaps the most fitting ending to this current volume. There are many questions left unanswered about the current state and future of the knowledge base of health promotion. Time will judge whether the current rate of change is disciplinary emergence, paradigm shift, or a less fundamental response to current changes in the policy environment. Philosophy may be the most appropriate subject from which to speculate on the possibilities for the future. This book is part of this speculation. It reviews the progress health promotion has made over the last twenty years or so by examining its disciplinary development. Clearly there are many disciplinary roots to health promotion theory and practice and in many ways this multi-disciplinarity is a strength.

Because it is a dynamic field, health promotion opens up exciting opportunities for both academics and practitioners to shape and determine the future direction of the discipline into the twenty-first century. What is already apparent is that the future of health promotion will involve increased theoretical development and debate to which the contributions in this volume are only a small part.

Robin Bunton
Gordon Macdonald
November 1991

REFERENCES

Arney, A. W. and Bergen, B. J. (1984) *Medicine and the Management of Living*, Chicago: University of Chicago Press.

Beattie, A. (1991) 'Knowledge and control in health promotion: a test case for social policy and social theory', in J. Gabe, M. Calnan, and M. Bury (eds) *The Sociology of the Health Service*, London: Routledge.

McQueen, D. (1991) *Health Education Research: Special Issue: Theory*.

Chapter 1

Health promotion
Discipline or disciplines?

Gordon Macdonald and Robin Bunton

Health promotion has emerged in the 1990s as a unifying concept which has brought together a number of separate, even disparate, fields of study under one umbrella. It has become an essential part of the new public health movement. Health promotion now forms an important part of the health services of most industrially developed countries and is the subject of a growing number of professional training courses and academic activities. The implications of this growth have concerned many of those involved in health and health care delivery. Some of the momentum for its development seems to have sprung from an increasing dissatisfaction with the bio-medical model or approach to health with its focus on disease, aetiology, and clinical diagnosis. There has been considerable interest in developing new approaches to health improvement. Less effort has been made, however, in considering the nature of this new form of knowledge and practice, its salient features and the likely constraints on and possibilities for its development.

This chapter is concerned with the recent, rapid development of discourse on health promotion as a field of study and practice. It asks whether or not health promotion may legitimately be thought of as a discipline and whether we can make sense of recent changes and conceptual ferment in terms of its emergence as a discipline. Though we argue that this question is far from answered, we suggest that recent changes in the knowledge base and the practice of health promotion are characteristic of paradigmatic and disciplinary development. The process and direction of development may not always be clear. Like the development of other bodies of knowledge, it can be complex and subtle. What is clear, however, is that a much broader range of theory is being drawn into the health promotion arena and alliances of theoretical approaches are being made. Different theories are being drawn upon in a variety of different practical orientations to produce a more varied practice. The knowledge base of health promotion would appear to be growing more multi-disciplinary, as the professional background of health promoters is becoming more varied. We might then conceive of this diversity and change as disciplinary and/or multi-disciplinary development.

Before considering this, it is valuable to review the nature of health promotion, its history, and how it relates to health education and public health.

WHAT IS HEALTH PROMOTION?

Health promotion represents at the very simplest level, whether one adopts a structuralist or individualist approach to health, a strategy for promoting, in some positive way, the health of whole populations. Definitions of health promotion abound (Tones 1983; WHO 1984; Tannahill 1985) but ultimately they all accept that both individual (lifestyle) and structural (fiscal/ecological) elements play critical parts in any health promotion strategy. These two main elements in health promotion give birth, in turn, to a number of subordinate themes. Essentially, lifestyle approaches are concerned with the identification and subsequent reduction of behavioural risk factors associated with morbidity and/or premature death.

But as one of the twin pillars supporting any health promotion strategy, the lifestyle element has a number of key subordinate themes grouped around the idea of education. Education involves the transfer of knowledge and skills from the educator to the student or learner. Knowledge improvement and attitude shift (cognitive and conative changes), health skills (behavioural changes), and the development of self-esteem are all constituent parts of these educational sub-themes. School health education curricula, stop-smoking clinics, and assertiveness training are all examples where these three educational methodologies are used in a lifestyle approach to health promotion. The structuralist strand also has a number of sub-themes. These centre around fiscal and legislative measures, such as alcohol taxation policies and seat-belt legislation, and ecological or environmental measures, such as new out-fall waste pipes near bathing beaches or the planting of more trees within an urban conurbation. Health protection measures such as screening and immunization programmes in a sense bridge the gap between the lifestyle approach and the structuralist approach, since both service provision and behaviour change are involved. Health promotion is concerned then with two principal themes and a number of subordinate themes all ultimately directed at reducing ill health and premature death. This view is not heterodoxy but now an accepted interpretation of conventional health promotion.

Conventional definitions of health promotion will continue, no doubt, to be characterized by diversity (Anderson 1984), even if recent conceptual developments are contributing to a convergence of views. Definitions of health promotion used by any one organization may be determined by political, social, and theoretical considerations; that is, the social context of an organization may well determine the approach to, and parameters around, health promotion, which makes any attempt at a universal definition almost impossible. It may be preferable to allow a certain elasticity of definition. Each definition might, reflexively, make explicit its position on fundamental issues, distinguishing itself from its competitors (Simpson and Issaak 1982). Different definitions can represent the different options or types of health promotion available to the health promoter according to the task or programme in hand. Definitions could then represent issues to do with health promotion goals, target populations, as well as the focus and type of intervention (Rootman 1985). Throughout this volume different notions of health promotion are being assumed, if not different conceptions of health. This may be seen as indicative of the current diversity of the field rather than any inherent flaw.

THE RISE OF THE NEW PUBLIC HEALTH

Health promotion did not grow in a vacuum but developed largely out of health education and in tandem with the development of the 'new public health' movement. This chapter is not concerned with a strict chronological development of health education since that is covered more than adequately elsewhere (Sutherland 1979), but it does give some space to the evolution of health promotion and its influence on the development of the new public health. Nor is it particularly concerned with the evolution of health promotion, at least not in an historical sense. It is concerned with how theory emerges and how theory influences, or indeed is influenced by, practice. We will refer to the different ways scientific knowledge and disciplines are developed and relate these to the recent shifts in theoretical reasoning underpinning much public health debate that have led to the development of health promotion.

Public health, if not medicine in general, has gone through a profound reorganization in the twentieth century. Nineteenth-century public health directed interventions, in the main, at environmental infrastructures that affected health. By the early twentieth century individual health had become a focus of concern, with the development of comprehensive vaccination and immunization programmes.

It is only in the second half of the twentieth century that we have witnessed a return to the more traditional nineteenth-century public health approaches with concerns about structure, environment, and ecology. A broader focus has become apparent within clinical medicine where the focus has been on the individual within his or her psycho-social context (Arney and Bergman 1984). Lifestyles and health behaviour have become concerns of public health and clinical medicine. Patients have been drawn into the diagnosis and treatment of disease. They have become not just consumers of health services but also quasi-producers of their health status. A theoretical shift reflecting these changes can be identified which undermines more traditional oppositions between health and illness (Armstrong 1988). Health promotion has emerged against this changing theoretical backdrop.

Health promotion first appeared as a term and concept in 1974 when the Canadian Minister of National Health and Welfare, Marc Lalonde, published *A New Perspective on the Health of Canadians* (Lalonde 1975). It introduced into public policy the idea that all causes of death and disease could be attributed to four discrete and distinct elements: inadequacies in current health care provision; lifestyle or behavioural factors; environmental pollution; and finally bio-physical characteristics. The basic message was that critical improvements within the environment (a structuralist approach) and in behaviour (a lifestyle approach) could lead to a significant reduction in morbidity and premature death. As a result of this report, the Canadian Government shifted its emphasis in public policy away from treatment to prevention of illness, and ultimately to the promotion of health. The Lalonde paper echoed the concerns of many who had become critical of a narrow view of health associated with the 'medical model'. Basaglia has expressed such sentiments, arguing that the medical model somehow separates the soma from the psyche, the disease from the patient, and the patient from the society in which he or she lives (Basaglia 1986). The roots of this model are said to lie in scientific explanations, aetiologies, clinical diagnoses and prognoses which ignore the far more complex social issues facing individuals in the world, such as employment (or unemployment), housing (or homelessness), and low income, or cultures engendering behaviour harmful to health.

The Lalonde report prompted a series of initiatives principally by the World Health Organization covering the next fifteen years or so and beginning with the Alma Ata declaration in 1977. This declaration, by the World Health Assembly at Alma Ata in the Soviet Union, committed all member countries to the principles of Health For All (HFA 2000). Although the principal thrust of the declaration was primary health care, it did incorporate a commitment to community participation and inter-sectoral action, now accepted elements within any serious health promotion programme. Implicit in the HFA strategy was this new vision of health promotion combining both lifestyle and structuralist approaches. WHO (Europe) launched its formal programme on health promotion using these twin supporting themes or pillars in 1984 (WHO 1984) and this programme gave rise to the first international conference on health promotion held in Ottawa, Canada, in November 1986.

The Ottawa conference concluded with the production of a charter which outlined five principal areas for health promotion action: building healthy public policy, creating supportive environments, strengthening community action, developing personal skills, and reorientating health services. These five action areas provide a useful framework for the delivery of health promotion programmes. The Ottawa Charter also included three process methodologies – mediation, enablement, and advocacy – through which people could begin to take control over their own health.

The second international conference on health promotion was held in Adelaide, Australia, in April 1988 and it concentrated more on healthy public policy as an arm of health promotion and delineated certain policy priorities. These were policies supporting the health of women, nutrition policies, policies on alcohol and tobacco, and policies concerned with the environment. Underpinning these priority areas were the twin concepts of health equity and policy accountability but also an implicit assumption that somehow only central government policy making had any real effect on measures for health promotion (WHO 1988).

The third international conference in Sandsvall, Sweden, in June 1991, focused on 'Supportive Environments for Health'. Specifically, it attempted to find practical ways to create physical, social, and economic environments for health compatible with sustainable development. It produced a handbook on action to improve public health and the environment (WHO 1991).

Health promotion then preceded the new public health movement, certainly etymologically if not epistemologically, though the two concepts are inextricably linked. Ironically, though, health promotion itself grew out of the legacy, albeit a narrow one, of health education. Sutherland (1979) points out that health education in the UK really started with the establishment of the Central Council for Health Education in 1927. This august body had two principal functions or aims: first, to 'promote and encourage education . . . in the science and art of healthy living' and, second, to 'coordinate the work of all statutory bodies in carrying out their powers and duties under the Public Health Acts . . . relating to the promotion . . . of Public Health'. Unfortunately health education confined itself in the main to the first, largely lifestyle, function and neglected the second, largely structuralist, issue. Health promotion in the last twenty years or so has attempted to fill that gap. It is worth noting, however, that health education in turn had not developed in a vacuum but had emerged as a consequence of the public health measures of the late nineteenth and early twentieth centuries.

Public health as a movement originated in the aftermath of the changes to the Poor Law with the Amendment Act of 1834. Edwin Chadwick was appointed to administer the new scheme and soon became aware that there was a relationship between poverty and ill health (Chave 1986). Sickness and ill health were largely the result of bad sanitation at home (and work) and filth and poor ventilation at work. As a result, Chadwick propounded his 'Sanitary idea' which was in effect the beginning of a national public health service, and gave rise to the first Public Health Act in 1848. John Simon took up Chadwick's ideas and as the first full-time salaried medical officer of health was instrumental in getting the second Public Health Act passed in 1872; this created local medical officers of health and led essentially to the medicalization of the public health movement. Although initially these doctors had a broad remit that included sanitation and housing, increasingly through the last quarter of the nineteenth century and the first quarter of the twentieth, they began to focus in on the bio-medical aspects of illness and disease which would later result in a lifestyle approach to public health. This was ultimately the reason for the setting up of the Central Council for Health Education in 1927. We can see then a dual development of health promotion and the new public health involving some interaction. Diagrammatically, this can be represented as follows:

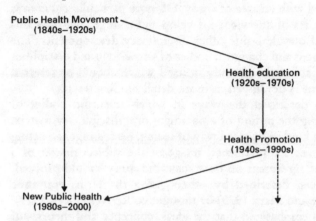

Public Health Movement
(1840s–1920s)

Health education
(1920s–1970s)

Health Promotion
(1940s–1990s)

New Public Health
(1980s–2000)

This typology plots the interdependent development of health promotion and the public health movement (old and new). Implicitly, it suggests that health promotion will contribute to, and form part of the new public health movement, contributing to the concepts used in public health and healthy public policy. Health promotion, characterized as a new body of expertise or 'new science' (McQueen 1988), has been informed by the rapid development of concepts and principles, largely, but not exclusively, derived from the social and behavioural sciences. Just as health education has been integrated and brought into health promotion (Tannahill 1985), it is suggested here that health promotion contributes to and becomes a part of the new public health. This 'new science' might continue to develop and identify diverse approaches to aetiology, assessment formulation, intervention, evaluation, and the analysis of the process of behavioural change. The growing influence and contribution of other disciplines within health promotion will contribute to the broader concerns of public health. Both individualist and structuralist perspectives within health promotion will also contribute to these broader concerns. This account of conceptual development draws largely upon developments in Europe and North America. Clearly concepts of health promotion in other parts of the world, and the south in particular, will vary (Morely *et al.* 1986). Discursive development in health promotion can, however, be seen to be heavily dependent upon work in the northern hemisphere.

DISCIPLINARY DEVELOPMENT AND CHANGE
Dictionary definitions of disciplines refer to their function to train or discipline scholars, introducing them to the 'proper action by instruction, exercising them in the same method and moral training' (*Shorter Oxford*

Dictionary 1985). A discipline then involves an ordered area or field of study, and it is this definition we use when we refer to disciplinary contributions to health promotion. In the context of this book, we are taking the term discipline to refer to bounded groups or federations of theories, perspectives, and methods associated with an area of study. Of more particular concern is how disciplines or bodies of knowledge develop and change, and how this development is carried out alongside other disciplinary developments. The nature of the development and change in bodies of knowledge and disciplines has become an identifiable field of study in itself which should be referred to here. (This argument is developed in more detail in Chapter 10.)

Thomas Kuhn has described the ways in which scientific bodies of knowledge change using the notion of a paradigm or a disciplinary matrix. A paradigm provides a kind of licensed way of seeing, describing, and acting upon the world. It gives a fundamental image of the subject matter of a discipline and levels of agreement on how scientific study should proceed. Such a notion has been described by others using the terms epistemic communities (Holzner and Marx 1979) or thought collectives (Fleck 1979). Like others, Kuhn has emphasized that the ideas, concepts, and theories of a scientific community are the outcome of collective effort and therefore subject to social and cultural influence. They will change and be transformed according to changes elsewhere in society. The routine grounds of scientific procedure are subject to change and modification. Kuhn draws our attention to periods of revolution and change, when the main features of the paradigm, those which order and organize a body of knowledge, undergo change.

Kuhn describes three basic stages of scientific development: a pre-paradigm stage in which several theories compete for dominance; a period of 'normal science' when a single paradigm has gained wide acceptance and provides the primary structuring of the field, and a crisis stage during which one paradigm is replaced by another. The development of physics can been used to illustrate this. Prior to Newtonian physics, there existed several competing systems of thought – the pre-paradigmatic stage. Newtonian thought provided a paradigm that replaced previous thought and provided an extended period of 'normal science'. This stage entered a period of crisis followed by the emergence of a new paradigm influenced by Einstein and Bohr (Kuhn 1962, 1970).

Kuhn's account suggests that once a revolution in thought has been achieved, it is followed by a more stable period in which the incremental growth typical of normal science is more usual. However, it is likely that the development of bodies of knowledge is more complex than this, involving, simultaneously, incremental growth as well as searches for new ordering principles that would restructure a paradigm. Moreover, many sciences or disciplines lack a single overarching paradigm and may be more accurately seen as multi-paradigmatic fields (Ritzle 1975). It is apparent that new ways of thinking frequently run alongside older systems, with a branching or segmented development (Holton 1973; Bucher and Stelling 1970). As different branches continue to develop, the boundaries of disciplines are permeated and new disciplines emerge.

Development of health promotion and the new public health can be seen to have occurred in this complex manner. More traditional concerns of public health and health education have run alongside the emergence and development of health promotion and the new public health. New objects of study, such as health behaviour, have emerged, whilst more traditional health education research has continued. New types of theories have been developed, drawing on different combinations of disciplines, or even new ones, whilst more traditional theory is still being used. We may be witnessing the emergence of new disciplines as well as the formation of new alliances of older ones. We can say that in recent years there has been increasing work directed at ordering the principles of public health and of health education/promotion. This work has resulted in considerable conceptual development characteristic of periods of paradigm change and revolution. It is probably also fair to say that this period of rapid theoretical and conceptual change is not yet over.

In referring to these developments we are not necessarily assuming such bodies of knowledge are sciences but merely that they show some similarities in their development and production. Knowledge production relating to areas of systematic organized enquiry has become increasingly important in the latter part of the twentieth century. The complex manner in which forms of knowledge are produced, organized, distributed, and applied are key features of what has been characterized as 'post-modern society' (Holzner and Marx 1979). Marked advances in information-handling capability, advanced communication techniques, and in particular the development of electronic information systems have changed the nature of social and institutional organization and have had a profound influence on our cultural system. The institutionalizing of technological knowledge and professional expertise has become a key social policy issue (Wilding 1982).

Nowhere is this more apparent than in health care where dependence upon highly differentiated specialized bodies of knowledge and specialized occupations or professions is at a premium. Health promotion has developed within the post-war period when the institutional structure of the health care delivery system, in the West at least, has grown dramatically in size and complexity. The development of bodies of knowledge surrounding health promotion, should be seen within this development and within the tendency towards systematizing of professional knowledge in general.

It may be possible to draw a distinction between the scholarly or scientific bodies of knowledge and the practising disciplines (Freidson 1970) as well as the professional groups that staff them. Most professional groups have made efforts to systematize, codify, and organize their bodies of knowledge. Not all would be considered as 'scientific' disciplines, though a move towards this hallowed status is discernible. The professional production of knowledge has developed arm in arm with the organization into disciplines within the university system, along with the production of a series of disciplinary ideologies. The health disciplines are no exception to this and their development may be viewed from within this system. Foucault's work has shed light on the history of human sciences, including medicine (Foucault 1970, 1973) and can be usefully drawn upon here. Analysing the emergence and development of a number of bodies of knowledge or 'discursive formations', he has identified a tendency towards systematization and self-reflection (Foucault 1973).

SCIENTIFICITY

Some discursive formations achieve what Foucault has called 'scientificity' (Foucault 1970). There is no inevitability about development towards this, and other types of systematized knowledge have emerged without subsequent development, yet still involving degrees of codification and formalization. There is no uniform, simple trajectory or evolutionary system as suggested by Kuhn (the authors' epistemological assumptions are in fact fundamentally different). Development is characterized by discontinuity and irregularity, dependent upon a number of social, political, and organizational forces. Forms of knowledge, Foucault argues, emerge within institutional arrangements and are subject to a complex number of influences. Because of this there are difficulties in distinguishing forms of knowledge and practice. In the public health field these distinctions are particularly difficult to make as the research and theoretical knowledge base has developed in interaction with health education/promotion practice. Practitioners have probably far outnumbered researchers and academics in the field. Moreover, this practice has been carried out by an extremely wide group of professions. The knowledge base has emerged (and is emerging) from a number of different sites. The emergence of psychopathology in France in Foucault's account shows some similarities with public health development (Foucault 1967).

The possibility of viewing objects of psychiatric investigation in eighteenth- and nineteenth-century France was dependent upon a whole number of conditions, including the existence of other discourses. Relationships between attendants of the insane and physicians, families, occupations, entrepreneurs, religious communities, and the local authorities all came to bear on the specific way psychotherapeutic concepts emerged. All these networks influenced the way people became classified as mad or sane.

In the eighteenth century this complex of forces allowed certain authorities to designate madness a legitimate object of enquiry. By the end of the nineteenth century medicine emerged as the dominant authority in delimiting this problem – though it was not the only one. It was primarily this medical authority which, by systems of referral, classification of behaviour and people, was able to build an institutional network that resulted in the development of asylums and attendant caring professions. The development of these institutions led to more clearly differentiated specification of the mad and sub-groups of the mad as well as appropriate treatment regimes.

The body of knowledge known as psychopathology, then, cannot be simply reduced to a gradually discovered set of objects of study to be conceptualized and classified. This knowledge was produced in mutual interdependence with the behaviour of families, the legal procedures, courts of law, and the mentally ill themselves. This analysis suggests ways of viewing the current development of the body of knowledge or discursive formation of health promotion.

To picture the emergence of health promotion as a body of knowledge, a discipline or set of disciplines, we must look to the institutions that practice and teach it, the professions that are involved in furthering its development, the political, social, and policy contexts in which it thrives or struggles, the different health cultures that exist to influence and draw upon it, as well as the bordering disciplines that feed, compete with, and influence its existence. A description of theoretical development within health promotion should take account of all of these features.

PROFESSIONAL IMPLICATIONS

Change in the knowledge base or paradigm of health promotion has been possible only through the efforts of those working within health promotion and public health. Equally, further change will have profound implications for those working in these fields. The structure of bodies of knowledge and the boundaries between different domains of study affect working experience, professional identity, and inter-professional relationships. Disciplines and bodies of knowledge are part of the major socializing mechanisms of the professions. Systems of selection, induction, graduation, and career channelling instil motivational commitments and forms of professional identity. Particular professional careers often possess their own distinctive heroic images and role models. Even within disciplines there may be sub-identities, associated with specific segments – medical sub-specialities being a case in point (Bucher and Stelling 1970).

The form of knowledge will mediate and regulate experience, identity, and working relationships, and, it follows, changes in this form of knowledge will change and disrupt these experiences, professional identities, and working relationships. Transmission of knowledge has specific effects. Modern concepts of health and disease, which underly the physician's role, are represented in the medical school curriculum, for example (Armstrong 1977; Atkinson 1981). Certain curricula invite strong professional allegiance by rigidly classifying the different subjects and allowing little cross-over between topics during training. Other curricula encourage the mixing of different disciplines and expect less subject or professional identity until later in careers. Bernstein (1971) has typified the English and the American education systems, respectively, in this way. Rigid division within a body of knowledge, such as medicine, psychiatry, or general practice, may reflect and perpetuate inter-professional differences.

The changes in conceptual structure within the new public health and health promotion fields will require a realignment of professional loyalties. The reorientation of health services referred to in the Ottawa Charter requires a reorientation in the ways health carers and promoters relate to one another. New working relationships and allegiances will need to develop to work to a new theoretical framework. New cross-disciplinary alliances may be formed to develop particular areas of study. Marketers, for example, may ally with public health medicine to work as social marketers. These new alliances will raise questions of professional identity. Are the doctors, nurses, psychologists, sociologists working in this field still identified as such or do they call themselves health promoters? Will courses in health promotion and public health stand as a post-qualification training or will they stand as a recognizable training in themselves? These questions bear on the nature of the development of health promotion as a discipline.

The current change and ferment in the health promotion field are suggestive of disciplinary development and formation. Alternatively, this development may be seen as part of a more general tendency towards multi-disciplinarity in the medical and other academic fields (Turner 1990). A feature of the new public health and of health promotion is a much broader focus than either public health or health education. A broader conception of the health field has been mentioned (Lalonde 1974; Green and Anderson 1986). With such a breadth of focus – human biology, environment, lifestyle, and health care organization – a broad disciplinary input is highly appropriate.

Social science has played a major, even cathartic role in developing the current range of concepts used, broadening the knowledge and practice base of health promotion. Sociology and psychology in particular have made significant contributions positing theories of behaviour related to health by reference to social constructs. Social psychological reasons for morbidity and individual health action have been put forward by some (Rosenstock 1974; Fishbein 1967; Festinger 1957; Bandura 1977), whilst explanations referring to social structures and macro-processes as determinants of health have been emphasized by others (Doyal 1979; Hart 1985; Aggleton 1990; O'Neill 1983; Donati 1988).

These social sciences have drawn the interest of other disciplines in health promotion, most notably education (Campbell 1985), economics (Maynard et al. 1989), and communication theory (Green 1980). These, along with sociology, psychology, and epidemiology, may be called primary feeder disciplines in that they have made a major and direct contribution to health promotion theory (and practice) but they are increasingly supported by secondary feeder disciplines whose contribution is at present less obvious. These would include philosophy, social policy, and marketing. All these primary and secondary feeder disciplines are given space in this book in an attempt to demonstrate the breadth of health promotion theory. They consolidate what for many has been a growing, even irritating, feeling that the bio-medical model of health promotion no longer offers an adequate explanation of why people think and behave the way they do.

Adoption of a multi-disciplinary approach to health promotion could avoid such a blinkered approach and may be more appropriate to the health issues of the late twentieth century. Multi-disciplinarity may be, in part, an answer to criticism aimed at bio-medically orientated health promotion. The current development of the knowledge base might be able to draw more fruitfully on feeder disciplines – primary and secondary.

SUMMARY

Health promotion is now an important and vital force in the new public health movement. Recent development in health promotion and public health has been rapid, fitting within broader shifts in medicine and health policy in the twentieth century. Within this change, health promotion may be seen to be developing both independently and in interaction with the new public health movement. Such rapid change is characteristic of paradigm shifts within bodies of knowledge and the emergence of new disciplinary alliances or even new disciplines. Given this, we might predict significant development of health promotion knowledge and practice along the lines of disciplinary formation. It is, however, too early to predict the outcome of this development. Disciplinary development is a complex and often subtle process and dependent on a large number of social, political, and inter-disciplinary factors. Moreover, paradigm shifts are not usually definitive or conclusive. More typically they occur along a continuum of change.

A lot can be at stake during periods of change. Professional power and identities are profoundly influenced by changes in their knowledge base. The appropriateness of a medical role in health promotion may continue to be debated. Issues of professional co-ordination and leadership may be discussed.

Adding to the complexity of current ferment within the health promotion field is the contribution to be made from a wide variety of disciplines. Whilst social science has played an important part in recent development, other disciplines also have a contribution to make. Another road for development is increased inter-disciplinarity within health promotion and public health. In which case the contributions from the variety of contributors to this volume will be especially relevant. If multi-disciplinarity is to be a feature of health promotion of the future, there is a need to consider the health promotion disciplines together in one volume.

REFERENCES

Aggleton, P. (1990) *Health*, London: Routledge.

Anderson, R. (1984) 'Health promotion: an overview', *European Monographs in Health Education Research* 6:1–126.

Armstrong, D. (1977) 'The structure of medical education', *Medical Education* 11: 244–8.

——(1988) 'Historical origins of health behaviour', in R. Anderson, J. Davies, I. Kickbusch, D. McQueen, and R. Turner (eds) *Health Behaviour Research and Health Promotion*, Oxford and New York: Oxford University Press.

Arney, W. A. and Bergman, B. J. (1984) *Medicine and the Management of Living*, Chicago: Chicago University Press.

Atkinson, P. (1981) *The Clinical Experience: The Construction and Reconstruction of Medical Reality*, Farnborough: Gower.

Bandura, A. (1977) *Social Learning Theory*, Englewood Cliffs, NJ: Prentice-Hall.

Basaglia, F. O. (1986) 'The changing culture of health and the difficulties of public health to cope with it', in *Vienna Dialogue on Health Policy and Health Promotion – Towards A New Conception of Public Health*, Eurosocial Research and Discussion Papers, European Social Development Programme.

Bernstein, B. (1971) 'On the classification and training of educational knowledge', in M. F. D. Young (ed.) *Knowledge and Control*, London: Collier Macmillan.

Bucher, R. and Stelling, A. (1970) 'Professions in process', in J. A. Jackson (ed.) *Professions and Professionalisation*, Cambridge: Cambridge University Press.

Campbell, G. (ed.) (1985) *New Directions in Health Education*, London: Falmer.

Chave, S. P. (1986) 'The origins and development of public health', *Oxford Textbook of Public Health*, Vol. 1, Milton Keynes: Open University Press.

Donati, P. (1988) 'The need for new social policy perspectives in health behaviour research', in R. Anderson, J. Davies, I. Kickbusch, D. McQueen, and D. Turner (eds) *Health Behaviour Research and Health Promotion*, Oxford and New York: Oxford University Press.

Doyal, L. (1979) *The Political Economy of Health*, London: Pluto.

Festinger, L. (1957) *A Theory of Cognitive Dissonance*, Stanford, CA: Stanford University Press.

Fishbein, M. (1967) 'Attitude and the prediction of behaviour', in M. Fishbein (ed.) *Readings in Attitude Theory and Measurement*, New York: Wiley.

Fleck, L. (1979) *Genesis and Development of Scientific Fact*, Chicago: University of Chicago Press.

Foucault, M. (1967) *Madness and Civilization*, London: Allen Lane.

——(1970) *The Archeology of Knowledge*, London: Tavistock.

——(1973) *The Birth of the Clinic*, London: Tavistock.

Freidson, E. (1970) *Profession of Medicine: A Study of the Sociology of Applied Knowledge*, New York: Dodd, Mead.

Green, L. W. (1980) *Health Education Planning: A Diagnostic Approach*, California: Mayfield.

Green, L. W. and Anderson, C. L. (1986) *Community Health*, 5th edition, St Louis, MO: Times Mirror/Mosby.

Hart, N. (1985) *The Sociology of Health and Medicine*, Ormskirk: Causeway Press.

Holton, G. (ed) (1973) *Modern Sciences and the Intellectual Tradition: Thematic Origins of Scientific Thought*, Cambridge, MA: Harvard University Press.

Holzner, B. and Marx, J. H. (1979) *Knowledge Application*, Boston, MA: Allyn & Bacon.

Kuhn, T. S. (1962) *The Structure of Scientific Revolutions*, Chicago: University of Chicago Press.

——(1970) *The Structure of Scientific Revolutions*, revised edition, Chicago: University of Chicago Press.

Lalonde, M. (1974) *A New Perspective on the Health of Canadians*, Ottawa: Information Canada.

McQueen, D. V. (1988) 'Thoughts on the ideological origins of health promotion', *Health Promotion*, Oxford: Oxford University Press.

Maynard, A., Godfrey, C., and Hardman, G. (1989) *Priorities for Health Promotion – An Economic Approach*, York: Centre for Health Economics, University of York.

Morley, D., Rohde, J., and Williams, G. (1986) *Practicing Health For All*, Oxford: University Press.

O'Neill, P. (1983) *Health Crisis 2000*, London: Heinemann.

Ritzle, G. (1975) *Sociology A Multiparadigm Science*, Boston, MA: Allyn & Bacon.

Rootman, I. (1985) 'Using health promotion to reduce alcohol problems,' in M. Grant (ed.) *Alcohol Policies*, Copenhagen: WHO.

Rosenstock, I. M. (1974) 'Historial origins of the health belief model', *Health Education Monographs* 2: 409–19.

Simpson, R. and Issaak, S. (1982) *On Selecting a Definition of Health Promotion: A Guide for Local Planning Bodies*, Toronto: Addiction Research Foundation.

Sutherland, I. (ed.) (1979) *Health Education Perspectives and Choices*, London: Allen & Unwin.

Tannahill, A. (1985) 'What is health promotion?', *Health Education Journal* 44(4):167–8.

Tones, B. K. (1983) *Education and Health Promotion: New Directions*, Institute for Health Education, Vol. 21, pp. 121–31.

Turner, B. (1990) 'The interdisciplinary curriculum: from social medicine to postmodernism', *Sociology of Health and Illness* 12(1):241–8.

WHO (World Health Organisation)(1984) *Health Promotion: European Monographs in Health and Health Education*, Research No 6, Copenhagen: WHO.

——(1985) *Health Promotion: A Discussion Document on the Concept and Principles*, Copenhagen: WHO.

——(1988) *The Adelaide Recommendations: Healthy Public Policy*, Copenhagen: WHO/EURO.

——(1991) *To Create Supportive Environments for Health. The Sundsvall Handbook*, Geneva: WHO.

Wilding, P. (1982) *Professional Power and Social Welfare*, London: Routledge & Kegan Paul.

Part I

Chapter 2

Psychology and health promotion

Paul Bennett and Ray Hodgson

The objectives of health promotion are necessarily diverse and complex, incorporating behavioural, social, environmental, political, and economic goals. This diversity of targets for change necessitates the use of a wide variety of applicable theory and practice. Often theories from several disciplines converge to focus on just one health outcome. Whilst psychological theories may claim no pre-eminence over other theories relating to health promotion, they nevertheless have a wide applicability because they attempt to explain behaviour and the mechanisms of change – both key aspects of health promotion work. Indeed, much early health education work was premised on psychological theories of mass communication developed in the 1950s and 1960s, in particular those developed at Yale.

These early theories assumed a relatively stable link between knowledge, attitudes, and behaviour. It was argued that if people were given appropriate information (i.e. smoking can damage your health) from an appropriate source (i.e. a doctor), this would change their attitudes towards smoking (i.e. 'I don't approve of smoking'), and in turn change behaviour (i.e. smoking cessation). However, the results of their primarily laboratory-based work often failed to replicate in more everyday settings. In particular, their assumption of a direct attitude–behaviour link has been strongly challenged by the relative ineffectiveness of programmes based on this premise and the parallel development of more sophisticated models of determinants of behaviour and behavioural change. Whilst in themselves open to criticism, these models may provide a better rationale for the development of health promotion programmes than the previous assumptions.

This chapter will, first, briefly describe some of the more recent theory used to explain the process of change in health-related behaviours. It will then introduce some worked examples of how these theories may be used to guide the development of health promotion programmes. Finally, it will present examples from three major heart disease prevention programmes of how these theories have been used in practice.

PSYCHOLOGICAL MODELS OF BEHAVIOUR AND BEHAVIOURAL CHANGE

The theory of reasoned action

Ajzen and Fishbein's (1980) theory of reasoned action attempts to make explicit the links between attitudes and behaviour. They argue that behaviour is governed by two broad influences. The first comprises the individual's attitudes towards a certain behaviour. Each attitude comprises a belief (e.g. smoking can cause cancer) and a valence attached to this belief (positive or negative) which may be strongly or more moderately felt. Individuals may have a number of conflicting attitudes towards a certain behaviour. Nevertheless, the sum of these various attitudes forms one source of influence on behaviour. The second source of influence, which they term subjective norms, are the individual's perceptions of what important others will think of their behaving in certain ways. These two major influences combine to form an 'intention' to behave in a certain manner, which is closely related to the behaviour itself. Thus the link between attitudes and behaviour is mediated by a number of processes each of which may influence behaviour.

These mediating links help explain why people do not always behave in accordance with their expressed attitudes. For example, an ex-smoker may have a number of negative attitudes towards smoking. However, they may smoke when out for a drink with friends who smoke as the subjective norms are that smoking is acceptable, even required, and drinking alcohol may interfere with a previous intention of not smoking. Equally, a person may jump out of an aeroplane attached to a flimsy bit of nylon or silk not simply because they have a positive attitude towards this behaviour (they may have an extremely *negative* attitude towards it at the point of exit from the aeroplane!) but because they do not wish to lose face with their friends; that is, go against the norms of the group they are in.

Social learning theory

A basic tenet of social learning theory (Bandura 1977; Hodgson 1984) is that behaviour is guided by expected consequences. The more positive these are, the more likely one is to engage in any particular behaviour. That said, many behaviours persist when what may seem negative consequences are likely to follow. A number of possible explanations for this paradox have been proposed. The first is simply that short-term gratification is more motivating than the prospect of long-term harm. For example, smokers may experience more short-term rewards for smoking in comparison to more nebulous, and potential, long-term negative consequences. Sometimes the consequences of an action are not actively imagined but simply lie dormant and, therefore, will not have a strong influence upon behaviour. Self-control involves activating and bringing to mind the longer-term consequences of our actions. Self-control, or self-regulation, is one of the aims of health promotion strategies.

Less obvious is the principle of *intermittent* reinforcement. Problem drinkers do not always derive satisfaction from drinking sessions; feelings of depression, anxiety, or violent aggression may be the outcome instead. Yet, on occasions, they do get the feeling of being at one with the world when alcohol transforms them into the gregarious, witty, and clever personality they would secretly like to be. Such outcomes may be very powerful determinants of future behaviour. A third explanation involves the notion of relativity of reinforcement. A smoker lighting up in a roomful of non-smokers may be acutely aware that his or her action is disapproved of. However, his or her justification is that they would feel even worse without a cigarette. The social discomfort they feel is easier to put up with than the discomfort of not smoking. Denial is another explanation of this paradox. A smoker who argues strongly that he or she knows a fit 92-year-old tobacco addict is using this example to offset their own subjective appraisal of the unhealthy consequences of smoking.

Social learning theory differentiates between *outcome* and *efficacy* expectations. Outcome expectancies refer to the consequences of an action (e.g. stopping smoking). Efficacy expectancies refer to the confidence that a person has in his or her ability to carry out an action or achieve a particular goal. Both types of expectancy have been shown to be related to the process of change.

One aspect of social learning theory has proven particularly important to health promotion – that is, the notion that one can learn behaviours and their outcomes through observation of others (vicarious learning). Skills learning is often conducted using direct observational learning. For example, budding heroin addicts are taught to prepare a syringe, find a vein, and 'mainline' the drug. Other types of drug users learn how to prepare their drugs for use, how to 'snort' cocaine or sniff glue, and what combination of drugs to use to achieve the best effect.

More indirect modelling of behaviour may come from watching television, films, and so on. Here a multitude of behaviours are shown with differing outcomes. These may or may not be appropriate or realistic. For example, alcohol consumption, often with few negative consequences, is over-represented on the television. This may suggest to young people that alcohol consumption is not only acceptable, but that the consequences are generally positive, thereby encouraging alcohol consumption.

There are individual differences in the degree to which people are influenced by modelling experiences, and not all models are equally influential. Under many circumstances, those models who have high status, competence, and power are more likely to influence the behaviour of the observer than a low-status model. For example, Lefkowitz *et al.* (1955), in a well-controlled experimental study, found that pedestrians were more likely to cross the street on a red light when they observed this behaviour from a high-status person in a pin-striped suit than when this transgression was performed by the same person dressed in patched trousers, scuffed shoes, and a blue denim shirt.

A further bias is related to the availability of evidence. People may have faulty beliefs regarding the outcomes of various behaviours simply because they are not exposed to a representative sample of the evidence. Slovic *et al.* (1976) have argued that this is the reason why people's beliefs about the most likely causes of death are so erroneous. Death from fire is usually considered to be more probable than death from drowning and accidental death more likely than death from a stroke, even though mortality figures strikingly show the opposite to be true. According to Slovic and his colleagues, this is because reports of fire and accidents are more likely to appear in the news media than accounts of death as a result of strokes and drownings.

Attribution theory

An important psychological factor which influences our ability to change is the reason, or causal attribution, we associate with a particular feeling or action. Attribution theory was used very ingeniously and fruitfully by Abramson *et al.* (1978) in their reformulation of the relationship between learned helplessness and depression. According to the original model, learning that unpleasant experiences cannot be controlled (learned helplessness) results in motivational, cognitive, and emotional deficits. The motivational deficit is reflected in passivity, intellectual slowness, and social impairment. The cognitive deficit consists of difficulty in re-learning that actions can control unpleasant experiences. The affective changes are a consequence of the expectation that bad outcomes are bound to occur since they cannot be controlled. The reformulation of the learned helplessness model is based upon the assumption that people not only experience helplessness, but that they also ask *why* they are helpless. In other words, they make a causal attribution. A woman whose child is having an appendix operation will experience a feeling of helplessness, but only until the child recovers. The helplessness does not generalize to many other areas and, furthermore, the experience is considered to be the result of external circumstances rather than personal inadequacies. This particular helplessness experience is attributed to transient, specific, and external events. On the other hand, a young man who performs badly at school and is dismissed from his first three jobs might easily conclude that there is something wrong with him which is an enduring characteristic and will hamper his progress in many areas of life. He is likely to attribute his helplessness to causes which are stable, global, and internal.

Health belief model

The health belief model (Becker 1974) was developed specifically to explain and predict behaviour in health contexts. While originally developed to predict preventive behaviours, the model has also been used to predict behaviour of both chronically and acutely ill patients. The model suggests that the likelihood of an individual engaging in a particular action is a function of their perceptions of the relationship between a behaviour and illness, their susceptibility to that illness, the seriousness of the illness, and the particular costs and benefits involved in engaging in the particular action. A final influence on the uptake of any behaviour is the presence of cues to action – that is, reminders to engage in certain behaviours. These various influences combine to determine behaviour, although the manner in which they combine to predict behaviour is imprecise.

Thus, an individual may be more likely to adopt a low fat diet if they are aware of the health consequences of a high fat diet and think that they are vulnerable to heart disease. Associated with such risk assessment is their belief as to whether the recommended diet will actually reduce their risk of heart disease.

The second process involves a cost/benefit analysis. In the case of dietary change the perceived benefits relate particularly to the long-term health benefits; that is, avoiding heart disease. The costs may be more immediate, and include changing cooking methods, eating less favoured foods, perhaps even an increase in the cost of shopping. It is therefore possible, even given the potential benefits, that the individual may decide it is not worth the effort to change. Finally, cues to action may help motivate or maintain behavioural change. These may include continued health warnings and advertising that emphasizes the health aspect of any product, labelling of food as low or high fat content, and so on.

Stages of change

Prochaska and DiClemente (1984) have analysed motivation to change across a wide range of problem areas and have identified five major stages of change. These are:

Precontemplation
Contemplation
Ready for action
Action
Maintenance.

At the *precontemplation* stage change is not being considered, whether through ignorance, denial, or demoralization. A young excessive drinker might consume the equivalent of five pints every night whilst drinking with his friends but does not believe that he has a drink problem. In the *contemplation* stage the same drinker might be perceiving a link between his marital problems and his alcohol consumption. Most people who are likely to be the targets of a health promotion initiative are in either the precontemplation or the contemplation stages. When perception of costs and benefits begins to alter a person might move into the *ready for action* stage and then into the *action* stage. The final stage, *maintenance*, occurs after a few months of successful action when attention is turned towards relapse prevention.

Evidence in support of this conceptualization is very strong. Motivation to change is along a dimension and is not all-or-nothing. Furthermore, progress through the stages is cyclical rather than linear. For example, most people attempting to stop smoking will relapse and find themselves back in the precontemplation stage. They become demoralized and do not want to consider a further attempt. Fortunately, the vast majority do eventually progress again to the contemplation and action stages. The measurement of stage of change is a very significant piece of information. For example, in one study of smokers, 20 per cent of precontemplators, 38 per cent of contemplators, and 67 per cent of those who were ready for action actually attempted to quit during the first six months of the study.

An important additional component of the stages of change model relates to processes of change. Prochaska and DiClemente identify the main processes and present evidence that different processes are relevant to the different stages. For example, raising awareness about the consequences of drug or alcohol abuse is a more appropriate intervention for drug users in the precontemplation stage. Coping skills training is more appropriate for those who are ready for action.

Communication theorists

A number of prominent workers have extended the original work of the Yale communication theorists to develop more sophisticated models of influence through mass communication. Some have focused on the optimum method of presenting information, but retained a model that continues to be predicated on the assumption that attitudinal change is sufficient to change behaviour. Others (e.g. McGuire 1984; Winett 1986) have become both more moderate in their claims for the outcome of mass communication and more eclectic in their methods. Thus Winett et al. (1989) are able to delineate a number of variables related to ineffective and effective information campaigns; note the change of goal to the provision of information, *not* behavioural change. These include high-quality production (even if limited exposure), targeted exposure, trustworthy, expert, and attractive sources, analysis of competing information to offset counter-argument, and so on. In addition they have drawn upon other theories, in particular social learning theory, to suggest how mass communication may provide a method of behavioural change through the use of modelling or vicarious learning principles.

As well as these considerations McGuire also emphasizes the need to understand target audience beliefs and perceived barriers to change before launching any campaign. This view is supported by Leathar (1981), who found that the key factors which affected young men's drinking in Glasgow was not the amount drunk on any one occasion – of which they did not keep a count (least of all in units) – but the time spent, and the social costs of, drinking. These factors, not health warnings related to units drunk per week (the intended campaign message), then became the focus of a media campaign. Similarly, Aggleton *et al.* (1987) found young men's beliefs relating to HIV transmission to be so far removed from the accepted medical model as to suggest that any health promotion message which simply described transmission routes would be unacceptable and unlikely to be acted upon by this population.

Diffusion theory

Diffusion theory (Rogers 1983; see also Chapter 9) moves from the primarily intra-individual processes involved in the previous models to consider a more societal model of change. It describes the dissemination of any innovation, such as new health-related behaviours, throughout society.

Typically, the entry and legitimization of an innovation, such as the uptake of a low fat diet, follows a characteristic S-shaped curve. Initial slow progress is followed by a rapidly increasing acceptance, with a final slowing as a late minority resist acceptance of the innovation. Different groups within the community are involved in different stages of the process. Early innovators provide a small initial 'foothold' for the innovation. These are, typically, high socio-economic status individuals and are often atypical of the community in which they live. Thus, their acceptance has little impact on the later diffusion of the innovation. However, they bring the innovation to the attention of a slightly more conservative group who are closer to the norms of the community, the so-called early adapters. The key phase in the introduction of a new innovation into the community is its acceptance by this group who are respected, have good communication systems, and are 'opinion leaders' within the community. If sufficient numbers accept the innovation, transmission and adoption are rapid through the community until only a minority of individuals fail to adopt the innovation, or do so only slowly.

Whilst a strong form of the model is difficult to assess, the model nevertheless brings to light a number of processes and issues particularly pertinent to preventive health interventions. Who are the opinion leaders who may influence the uptake of health-related behaviours? What are the dynamics of opinion leading? Can these opinion leaders become a resource for any community intervention? How can appropriate behaviours be maintained in the face of subsequent innovations? and so on. One, rather adverse, implication of the model is that if early adopters are sufficiently deviant from societal norms, this may slow or even prevent the spread of the innovation to the rest of the population. For example, it is possible that early adoption of condom use by homosexual men may have acted to inhibit use by those who do not wish to be identified with this particular group.

PUTTING THE THEORIES TO WORK

The theories described above attempt to explain behaviour and behavioural change. Clearly, none provides a full explanation of the adoption or failure to adopt health behaviours. However, they do suggest key variables that may interact to predict behaviour, and we would argue that a synthesis of the models may provide a strong basis to any health promotion initiative targeted at individual behaviour change. Thus, rather than treat them as abstract theories, we will attempt to show in the next section how they may collectively provide differing frameworks around which to plan a health promotion intervention.

Example 1: developing an AIDS programme

Transmission of HIV is almost exclusively through individually determined behaviours: sexual intercourse and the use of intravenous (IV) drugs. As such, HIV/AIDS presents a major challenge to all involved in health promotion (in its widest sense) as control of the spread of the virus can primarily be brought about through understanding and influencing the behaviour of key groups within the population. The theories outlined above may help prevent the spread of HIV in two ways: first, by providing some insight into factors that influence 'risky' behaviours and, second, by providing some pointers to how these factors may be modified. These two issues are examined below, with particular regard to the adult population.

Understanding behaviours

One of the more difficult groups to influence in any HIV/AIDS campaign has been IV drug users. It is easy to suggest that this is because they form some 'deviant' group that is insensitive to health promotion messages. An alternative perspective would suggest that a variety of factors combines to make appropriate behaviour change difficult – that is, inappropriate in the contexts of these people's lives.

Needle and syringe ('works') sharing still remains the main route of HIV infection in IV drug users, despite their apparently high levels of knowledge about the virus and its modes of transmission. Clearly factors other than knowledge of risk are affecting behaviour. One major reason, in the absence of needle exchange schemes, is simply the lack of clean needles. However, an important function of sharing the 'works' is that this lowers the risk of being caught by the police. Sharing also carries a social function, as many users share needles with partners or (less frequently) friends. Thus, both the cost-benefit pay off and social norms support the maintenance of needle sharing. The perceived risks of participating in needle exchange schemes may also mean that their use will be low until some confidence is established in their safety. Finally, drug users' perceptions of risk may differ markedly from other groups'. They already undertake highly risky behaviour – indeed the risks associated with drug use may be one of its attractions. Thus the risk of disease may confer little further anxiety, or even enhance the thrill.

When considering sexual behaviour, again the constraints on the adoption of safer sex practice, particularily the use of condoms, are high. To a generation brought up with non-disruptive contraception their use does not come easy. Equally, there are the problems in purchasing them and introducing the subject during any pre-sexual preamble with a new partner. Each produces the potential for embarrassment and difficulties, particularly when an individual has poor social skills or little practice in discussion of such matters. Thus when the perceived threat of infection is low, the cost/benefit equation may fall on the side of unsafe sexual practices, particularly when the perceived norm remains unprotected sex.

Changing sexual behaviours

The mass media, whilst not in themselves sufficient to bring about widespread behavioural change, nevertheless provide an entry point to any health promotion campaign related to HIV. A sophisticated campaign should do more than simply provide information relating to risk and risk reduction. Information needs be phased and interrelated to other aspects of any campaign, and opportunities should be used to model appropriate behaviours as well as to teach skills necessary for the uptake of behaviours.

Critical to the first stage of any campaign is the provision of accurate and *relevant* information to those at risk. Individuals need be aware of their *personal* risk of HIV infection, the severity of the implications, and (critically) what they can do to reduce or eliminate their personal risk. It is neither necessary nor sufficient to use deliberate highly fear-arousing campaigns such as the iceberg campaign in the UK or the grim reaper campaign in Australia. These evoke high levels of anxiety, yet provide no means of reducing that anxiety and do not bring about behavioural change.

Whilst some information on AIDS/HIV and preventive behaviours (e.g. use of condoms, safer sex) may be necessary for the community in general, some information (e.g. regarding sexual practices, availability of needle exchange schemes) may be inappropriate or offensive to the wider public. Information channels should therefore be targeted so that appropriate information is made available to all the relevant groups, for example, through local or specialist radio, street workers, specialist press (gay, music), and so on. The value of leaflets providing specific, explicit, and targeted information must also be recognized.

The week-long BBC and ITV scheduling of AIDS educational material provided a good model of how information relating to risk and required behavioural change may be undertaken. This campaign was influential as it not only told people that certain behaviours were necessary, it actually showed (modelled) how to perform them, for example by giving explicit demonstrations of how to put a condom on. The programmes indulged in a fair degree of humour, again providing a model of safer sex that is fun rather than merely mechanical, and were often presented by role models liked and respected by the target audience, including youth television and radio presenters. In addition, there were a number of studio discussions conducted by young people which aimed to dispel ignorance or myths surrounding sexual practice and HIV infection, helping offset any counter-arguments to change.

Whilst the campaign had a number of strengths, it had two significant weaknesses; it was too brief to respond to changing public opinion and behaviour and it did not provide later cues to action necessary to maintain behavioural change. These refinements are developed in a model programme suggested by Winett et al. (1989), aimed at increasing condom use. As a first phase, they suggest a wide-ranging information campaign accompanied by free distribution of condoms. At the same time they suggest the development of a lottery, based on numbers available on condom covers, to directly reinforce the use – or at least the purchase – of condoms. Explicit instruction in the use of condoms could also be given through the mass media and at the points of distribution (e.g. schools, community sites). Critical to their intervention is the appropriate use of modelling during a series of television spots. They suggest models may be initially sceptical of condoms but 'after appropriate segues and scenes' they could move to a position in which they can say how using a condom increases their spontaneity and pleasure because they know they are safe. They advocate measurement of the uptake of condoms as a measure of the success or failure of the campaign, allowing later fine-tuning of the campaign (for example, by placing greater emphasis on the value of both men and women carrying condoms).

The media may also play a more subtle role. Popular soap operas have already been used to portray in an acceptable light the problems of homosexuality in relation to AIDS (EastEnders, BBC television) and drug addiction (Brookside, Channel 4 television, UK). Such influences are unfortunately all too rare, and often inappropriate images are given. In particular, sex is almost universally portrayed as exciting, free spirited, and free from such hassles as condoms and safer sexual practice. Such a deficit has two major disadvantages. First, it provides a source of normative influence that is inappropriate – 'no one else uses a condom, why should I?'. In addition, by providing an inappropriate model of 'how to do sex', the media also fail to provide vicarious learning experiences of 'how to do sex *properly*'. Whilst the use of condoms, introduction of safer sex practices, and prior discussion are delicate issues for the writer and producer, if sexual behaviours are to be portrayed on the television and cinema, such issues need to be explored. In America a consulting service led by a psychologist and scriptwriter has provided advice to producers on how to portray less alcohol consumption in a number of popular soap operas. Perhaps now is the time to develop a similar service relating to other health issues.

Whilst the media have a potentially powerful role to play in the prevention of the spread of HIV, it must be remembered that there are a multitude of other influences on behaviour. These may be structural, relating to the provision of services (education or health), or environmental. For example, local voluntary agencies may be the best providers of personalized advice concerning AIDS/HIV and safer sexual practice, or distributing leaflets, explicit videos, etc. Any such service should be specialist and, where possible, involve key members (opinion leaders) of appropriate communities. They will have the advantage of speaking the same language as users and providing strong role models. It is also important that any service should not simply form a crisis function, but be widely and freely available to act as advisers on sexual practice, provide help in developing appropriate social skills, and so on.

Other, more environmental, changes may also promote appropriate behaviours. One key, and potentially embarrassing, aspect of safer sex has nothing to do with the sexual act itself – it is the purchase of condoms. The most radical approach to encouraging their use may be to make them freely available to all potential users (as indeed they are to attenders at Family Planning Clinics). Other approaches may involve making their sale more easily and less embarrassingly accomplished; for example, by selling them at a price rounded up or down (i.e. £1 versus £1.15) to avoid the necessary wait for change. Alternatively, more widespread distribution through supermarkets may normalize their use and make purchase simpler. Finally, as women are encouraged to take more responsibility for their own protection (both from HIV and pregnancy) it is important to increase the availability of condoms to women, for example by selling them in women's toilets.

One final approach relates to cues to action. It is noticeable that news relating to AIDS and the spread of HIV varies in concentration, and, as it does so, so does public concern. There is also some evidence that even people who begin to take up safer sex practices may 'relapse' over time. Thus, cues to action need to be continually provided (as well as repeated information campaigns), emphasizing the positive aspects of safer sexual practice. These may include advertising of condoms, articles relating to sexual practice in key magazines, theatre workshops, displays, and so on.

Example 2: developing a 'sensible drinking' programme

The psychological models which have been outlined in this chapter are applicable to the early experimentation with alcohol and subsequent social drinking, as well as the development of a drinking habit and dependence. This section will focus upon just two possible health promotion responses to excessive drinking: self-regulation approaches directed towards early identification and early intervention, and community responses aimed at modifying the social environment to alter the balance of incentives and barriers to consumption.

Self-regulation

Self-regulation, or self-control, skills have been investigated by psychologists in a wide range of settings and problem areas. In fact, self-regulation theory is one way of integrating some of the concepts and theories described earlier (Miller and Brown, in press). One specific counselling approach, usually called self-control training, has been used to help problem drinkers. Typically, this educational or counselling course would be spread over ten sessions and achieves very good results for moderately dependent drinkers aiming for a controlled drinking goal.

In order to investigate even lower cost alternatives Miller and his colleagues carried out a further piece of research which is very relevant to a health promotion perspective (Miller and Taylor 1980). This study demonstrated that a self-help manual which teaches a self-control approach turns out to be as effective as ten sessions of training carried out by an experienced therapist. Furthermore, these findings have been consistent across populations varying widely in socio-economic and educational status. A more recent UK study has also confirmed the usefulness of a self-help manual (Heather et al. 1986).

Miller and Sanchez (in press) have reviewed a number of studies which have demonstrated the effectiveness of brief interventions in reducing alcohol consumption and problems. They summarized the common components of these studies using the acronym FRAMES which stands for: Feedback, Responsibility, Advice, Menu, Empathy, and Self-efficacy. The assessment of health and social status followed by *feedback* of results is included as a key component in most brief interventions. The feedback could be of liver functioning or of the possible link between excessive drinking and sexual, marital, social, or work problems. Personal *responsibility* for change is emphasized. The aim is to promote internal attributions of responsibility for change rather than encouraging a reliance on external agents and a sense of helplessness. *Advice* to change is a third common element. Advice given sensitively by a high status or respected person can be 'a cue to action' and move a person from one stage of change to the next. Sometimes, advice to change is accompanied by a *menu* of specific recommendations from which to chose. The counsellor or change agent's ability to *empathize* with a problem drinker has been shown to be important and the development of *self-efficacy* expectations is of crucial importance.

These components are clearly those which would be suggested by the various theories described earlier. The focus upon feedback of results in an attempt to modify outcome and efficacy expectancies would be at the heart of an intervention derived either from social learning theory, the theory of personal action, or the health belief model. Attribution theory leads to the prediction that the process of change is facilitated by taking personal responsibility for change rather than relying upon continuous help from others. The advice is always given by a relatively high status person (e.g. doctor, psychologist, nurse) within appropriate sectors (e.g. hospital or health centre). In other words the cue to action is given by an 'expert' at a time when the relationship between excessive drinking and health is a matter of concern and the drinker is more likely to be moving from contemplation to action.

The proven effectiveness of brief interventions is an important finding which health promoters are taking on board. It changes the way in which we view a comprehensive treatment service. Instead of using scarce resources to proliferate hospital treatment units, the first priority must be to ensure that each community has a widespread network of low-cost interventions. These could be based within a primary care setting, a community alcohol team, a community mental health centre, or a district general hospital out-patient department. Pamphlets and manuals should be easily available from health centres, social services, pharmacists, and other centres involved in providing help. The main objective of an alcohol service should be to ensure that it is relatively easy to get some advice and support directed towards changing outcome and efficacy expectancies. Higher-cost alternatives would then be developed only for clients who require more intensive help and only when there is good evidence that such approaches are likely to be effective.

Community responses

Screening procedures designed to identify early drinking problems will not reach the large number of people within most societies who are drinking in a hazardous way but are not yet experiencing problems. A comprehensive health promotion approach involves many strands but one major component is to encourage a large number of people and groups to change their attitudes, policies, and actions in order to make healthy choices easier and more probable (see Robinson *et al.* 1989). As examples, reference will be made to two investigations which strongly suggest that excessive drinking is a behaviour which can be influenced by ensuring that there are 'cues to action' at the very moment when a drinker is ready to consume more.

The two studies demonstrate the following principles:

1   Health promotion is often concerned with changing the attitudes and actions of those people or organizations in a position to influence behaviour (e.g. police, publicans).
2   The same concepts or theories of change that have already been discussed apply equally when attempting to move those people from precontemplation to action.

The first investigation is based upon the hypothesis that the police can have a powerful preventive influence on drink-related problems simply by reminding both the publican and the drinker that excessive drinking can be illegal. Jeffs and Saunders (1983) were able to evaluate the effectiveness of a community policing strategy which was implemented in an English seaside resort during the summer of 1978 and then withdrawn the following year. Public houses in the harbourside area of the town were visited by two police-men and the first step was to remind licensees of their responsibilities under the licensing legislation. The licensees and the police agreed to co-operate fully in an attempt to ensure that the law was observed, particularly as it relates to under-age drinking and serving alcohol to those who are already intoxicated. During the summer months the selected premises were then visited regularly. Two or three uniformed officers amicably, but very conspicuously, checked for under-age drinking or the presence of persons who were the worse for drink. The checking was very thorough and was designed to bring home to both staff and patrons the seriousness of their intention to enforce the licensing laws and, incidentally, bring the costs of such drinking to salience for both drinkers and publicans.

In order to test the effectiveness of this preventive exercise the rates of recorded crime and public order offences for the summer of 1978 were compared with those for the year before as well as the year after. Such an analysis did indeed suggest that crime in 1978 was 20 per cent less than would be expected from an extrapolation of the figures for 1977 and 1979. The implication that this change resulted from the alteration in police practice is supported by two additional pieces of evidence. First, this result was not apparent in a control town within the same tourist region. Second, the reduction in 1978 was greater for alcohol-related crimes than for those, such as burglary and theft, which are not strongly related to alcohol consumption.

This study, carried out by a psychologist and a policeman, suggests that a comparatively minor change in police practice, albeit a major change in policy, produced results which would be quite dramatic if they could be replicated throughout the world. There were 2000 fewer arrests in the experimental year than would be expected. This is not a trivial outcome.

The second study also focuses upon ways of influencing alcohol consumption in the setting of a public bar (Geller *et al.* 1987). This American investigation looked at the effectiveness of an intervention, usually called server training, designed to help servers to identify customers who are about to drink excessively. The training then covers a variety of tactics for dealing with such customers: for example, offering food or alternative drinks, or discussing the catastrophic consequences that can result from drinking and driving. Seventeen servers of alcohol and thirty-two research assistants participated in the study, the latter visiting the servers' place of work and posing as customers in order to provide double-blind before and after assessments. The pseudo-customer attempted to consume one drink every twenty minutes but they could be influenced by the server intervention strategies. All interactions between the servers and the pseudo-customers were recorded independently by other assistants. The results of the study were quite clear. Trained servers intervened more regularly and appropriately compared to the same servers prior to training, as well as a control group of untrained servers. The blood alcohol concentration of pseudo-customers was also assessed as they left the bar. Prior to the training 37.5 per cent of the pseudo-customers left the bars legally drunk. In contrast no pseudo-customer served by a trained server reached the legal limit of intoxication.

These studies of community policing and server training modify both social setting and expectancies regarding the costs and benefits of drinking at that crucial moment when a decision is being made about future alcohol consumption. Together, they suggest that alcohol consumption can be influenced at the point of sale and that health promotion and crime prevention resources should be channelled into similar projects.

Interventions by the police, publicans, and servers might be expected to reach the very large numbers of hazardous drinkers who are not reached by screening strategies directed at the early problem drinker. The most important consideration is whether a large number of chief constables and publicans can be persuaded to take on such a health promotion or prevention role. Community policing tends to suffer when resources are stretched. Furthermore, many policemen are not happy with such a role ('I didn't join the police force to be a social worker'). We are at a very early stage in the diffusion of these ideas throughout society. Certainly a number of chief constables, publicans, and magistrates have become the early innovators. The media focus upon drunk-driving as well as alcohol and violence provides the ideal background for the rapid diffusion of these strategies. Nevertheless, whether the police and publicans adopt them in large numbers will depend upon their own perception of outcome and efficacy expectancies, their causal attributions, and the models they are exposed to.

A comprehensive community response must involve collaboration between magistrates, licensees, alcohol advisory committees, health and social services, education, trade unions, and the voluntary sector. The basic aim of a community strategy is to make healthier choices easier by changing outcome and efficacy expectancies.

CASE STUDIES IN HEART DISEASE PREVENTION

Coronary heart disease (CHD) has been an important focus for health promotion for three reasons. First, it is the most widespread cause of premature death, at least in the developed world. Second, risk for disease can be modified by personal action: diet, smoking, exercise levels, and so on are all, at least to some extent, individually determined. Finally, there is strong evidence that a large percentage of the population is at risk due to one or more risk factors. Thus, if behaviour is modifiable using health promotion methods, a large percentage of the population will have health benefits from making appropriate behavioural changes. Heart disease prevention programmes have formed some of the largest and most sophisticated attempts at health promotion. Most of the major programmes have been explicitly premised, at least in part, on the models discussed in this chapter. The final section will thus examine how they have guided interventions, and with what effect.

Although not the largest programmes, the North Karelia Project in Europe and the Stanford Three City Project in North America are perhaps the two which have been most carefully evaluated. Both involved media- and community-based interventions. The Stanford Project (Maccoby 1988) compared the effects of an intensive media campaign, alone or in combination with intensive counselling of high-risk individuals, with a no-intervention control in three comparable Californian towns. Two towns became the focus of a year-long media campaign providing information about heart disease and ways of reducing personal risk. A number of subjects in one town found to be at high risk of disease also received group or individual counselling on diet, smoking, and exercise. A third town received no intervention.

Social learning and communication theory suggested the content and timing of the media output: first, to provide information and motivate behavioural change; next, to demonstrate behavioural change; and, finally, to model and cue new behaviours. Models were seen coping effectively with change, such as going through a smoking cessation group or having a family picnic using 'healthy food'. Social learning principles also provided the underpinning of the intensive individual interventions. A natural extension of the intensive counselling interventions was the development through social networks of a diffusion system of skills and information gained in the groups.

The North Karelia Project (Puska *et al.* 1985) used similar approaches to the Stanford study. Social learning theory, the theory of reasoned action, and communication theories explicitly governed timing, distribution, and content of a five-year media and health education campaign. Attention was given to appropriate modelling, suppressing counter-arguments, modifying social norms, and providing the skills necessary for change. For example, much was made of the fact that the recommended diet was in fact more traditional than their present high fat diet; a vegetarian athlete was used as an example to show that eating meat was not the only way to be fit and healthy. Just as in Stanford, television programmes showed how 'ordinary' people gave up smoking. Environmental contingencies were also set up to enhance or maintain behaviour change; for example, shops were encouraged to display 'No smoking' signs, low fat sausages were produced at a local sausage factory, and the county dairy actively promoted low fat products. Diffusion theory provided the basis for the use of lay opinion leaders in attempting to spread knowledge of ways of reducing personal risk of CHD. Media and education programmes were not the only vehicle for promoting change. Specific instruction or help could be gained at local colleges, sports clubs, and women's societies for people wishing to give up smoking or change their diet. Finally, local medical services took on a more preventive role.

These programmes operated at a town or county level. But it is possible to organize interventions at a more local or wider level – or indeed to combine both. Heartbeat Wales (Nutbeam and Catford 1987) focused on a total population of nearly three million and organized interventions primarily through the development of local networks as well as using the mass media. This project had many commonalities with the previous projects, but also had some innovative differences, particularly in relation to environmental factors. In particular, it worked with food manufacturers and distributors to promote food labelling (low fat, low sugar) and the selling of healthy foods, including low fat meat cuts and so on. In addition, it encouraged the development of 'healthy eating' schemes (low fat choices, no smoking areas) in both the workplace and restaurants. They also negotiated with public houses to encourage the sale of low alcohol drinks and to negotiate non-smoking bars. Thus, they established a number of cues to action and made appropriate behavioural choice easier than it may have been previously (i.e. reduced the costs of behavioural change).

How effective have these programmes been in bringing about change? The signs appear to be good. Both the Stanford and North Karelia projects found reductions in risk factors and/or morbidity to heart disease following the intervention (Heartbeat Wales has still to report its findings). However, evaluating the effectiveness of these interventions has proven exceptionally difficult, and appropriate methodologies are still being developed. Thus, we are still unable to prove an *unequivocal* link between any intervention and changes in behaviour and morbidity. To give one illustration. The Stanford Project followed a cohort of subjects throughout the life of the project to determine whether they had made any behavioural changes. Unfortunately, knowing that they formed part of a research project – and having learned what they 'should' be doing – some subjects apparently changed their behaviour before they were assessed. For example, some subjects who knew they were going to have their serum cholesterol measured made appropriate dietary changes (only) in the weeks before their appointment. To obviate such problems, the North Karelia Project measured risk factors and behaviour in three *different* groups of individuals over the course of the study, and found a number of changes in risk behaviour and morbidity for CHD. However, they ran into problems of a different sort. It is possible that changes in diet and smoking may have reflected improvements in living standards in North Karelia during the time of the project. In addition, an influx of city dwellers over the period of the project may have meant that the samples studied at each time contained increasing numbers of incomers – each bringing a different lifestyle unrelated to the project. Thus the changes found may simply reflect the changes in population and not an effect of the intervention. It's not easy being a researcher on these projects!

CONCLUSIONS

Psychological theory can provide a key underpinning to health promotion theory and programmes at all levels of intervention. Sometimes theory may simply provide a strong rationale for what may seem an obvious and logical intervention. On other occasions, theory may provide something of more substance. In both cases, arguably, they help bring order to an abundance of potential interventions, and in doing so impose some logic on any complex health promotion programme. Of course, psychological theories are constantly developing and changing – indeed, application of theories to health promotion is helping such developments. Other models may supersede or combine with those described here (see for example Bunton *et al.* in press) to make health promotion more effective in the future. It must be to the advantage of both health promoters and psychologists to develop theory and practice in tandem, to better inform future health promotion programmes, and to improve the public health.

REFERENCES

Abramson, L. Y., Seligman, M. E. P., and Teasdale, J. D. (1978) 'Learned helplessness in humans: critique and reformulation', *Journal of Abnormal Psychology* 87: 49–74.
Aggleton, P., Homans, H., and Warwick, I. (1987) 'Health education, sex and AIDS', paper presented at the International Society of Education Conference, Birmingham.
Ajzen, I. and Fishbein, M. (1980) *Understanding Attitudes and Predicting Behaviour*, Englewood Cliffs, NJ: Prentice-Hall.
Bandura, A. (1977) *Social Learning Theory*, Englewood Cliffs, NJ: Prentice-Hall.

Becker, M. H. (1974) 'The health belief model and personal health behaviour', *Health Education Monographs* 2: 324–508.

Bunton, R., Murphy, S., and Bennett, P. (1991) 'Theories of behavioural change and their use in health promotion', *Health Education Research, Theory and Practice* 6:153–62.

Geller, E. S., Russ, N. W., and Delphos, W. A. (1987) 'Does server intervention training make a difference? An empirical field evaluation', *Alcohol, Health and Research World* 2(4): 64–9.

Heather, N., Whitton, B., and Robertson, I. (1986) 'Evaluation of a self-help manual for media recruited problem drinkers: six-month follow-up results', *British Journal of Clinical Psychology* 25: 19–34.

Hodgson, R. J. (1984) 'Craving and priming', in G. Edwards and J. Littleton (eds) *Pharmacological Treatments for Alcoholism*, London: Croom Helm.

Jeffs, B. and Saunders, W. (1983) 'Minimising alcohol-related offences by enforcement of the existing licensing legislation', *British Journal of Addiction* 78: 67–77.

Leathar, D. S. (1981) 'Lack of response to health guidance amongst heavy drinkers', in M. R. Turner (ed.) *Preventive Nutrition and Society*, London: Academic Press

Lefkowitz, M., Blake, R. R., and Moulton, J. S. (1955) 'Status factors in pedestrian violation of traffic signals', *Journal of Abnormal Social Psychology* 51: 704–5.

Maccoby, N. (1988) 'The community as a focus for health promotion', in S. Scapapan and S. Oskamp (eds) *The Social Psychology of Health*, Newbury Park, CA: Sage.

McGuire, W. J. (1984) 'Public communication as a strategy for inducing health-promoting behavioural change', *Preventive Medicine* 13: 299–319.

Miller, W. R. and Brown, J. M. (in press) 'Self regulation as a conceptual basis for the prevention and treatment of addictive behaviors', in N. Heather, and W. R. Miller and J. Greely (eds) *Self Control and the Addictive Behaviors*, Oxford: Pergamon.

Miller, W. R. and Sanchez, V. C. (in press) 'Motivating young adults for treatment and lifestyle change', in G. S. Howard (ed.) *Issues in Alcohol Use and Misuse by Young Adults*, Notre Dame, IN: University of Notre Dame Press.

Miller, W. R. and Taylor, C. A. (1980) 'Relative effectiveness of bibliotherapy, individual and group self-control training in the treatment of problem drinkers', *Addictive Behaviours* 5: 13–24.

Nutbeam, D. and Catford, J. (1987) 'The Welsh Heart Programme: progress, plans and possibilities', *Health Promotion* 2: 5–18.

Prochaska, J. O. and DiClemente, C. C. (1984) *The Transtheoretical Approach: Crossing Traditional Foundations of Change*, Homewood, IL: Don Jones/Irwin.

Puska, P., Nissinen, A., Tuomilehto, J., Salonen, J. T., Koskela, K., McAlister, A., Kottke, T. E., Maccoby, N., and Farquhar, J. W. (1985) 'The community-based strategy to prevent coronary heart disease: conclusions from the ten years of the North Karelia Project', *Annual Review of Public Health* 6: 147–93.

Robinson, D., Tether, P., and Teller, J. (eds) (1989) *Local Action on Alcohol Problems*, London: Routledge.

Rogers, E. (1983) *Diffusion of Innovations*, New York: The Free Press.

Slovic, P., Fischoff, B., and Lichtenstein, S. (1976) 'Cognitive processes and societal risk-taking', in J. S. Carroll and J. W. Payne (eds) *Cognition and Social Behaviour*, Hillside, NJ: Lawrence Erlbaum.

Winett, R. A. (1986) *Information and Behaviour: Systems of Influence*, Hillsdale, NJ: Lawrence Erlbaum.

Winett, R. A., King, A. C., and Altman, D. G. (1989) *Health Psychology and Public Health*, New York: Pergamon Press.

Chapter 3

What is the relevance of sociology for health promotion?

Nicki Thorogood

INTRODUCTION

This chapter will be considering how sociology can contribute to both the theory and the practice of health promotion. It is my contention that many sociological categories are implicit in the work of health promotion and that articulating them can only improve our knowledge and how we use it. The chapter falls into four main sectors. The first, 'What is sociology?', offers a short introduction to the main theoretical approaches of the discipline and to its key concepts. Clearly space here is limited and I would recommend any interested students to refer to more comprehensive introductory texts. The second section, 'Sociology of health and illness', briefly considers the role of the discipline in the field of health and illness. This charts its development from being in the service of medicine, to analysing the professional organization of medicine; to incorporating the perspectives of 'ordinary' people; to its present position of providing a critique of medical knowledge and practice.

The third and fourth sections address themselves in more depth to the project of health promotion. The first of these, 'Sociology as applied to health promotion', considers the ways in which a sociological perspective can aid the work of health promotion. It takes some of the accepted categories of sociology – lay beliefs, social stratification, gender, age, and race – and shows how sociological analysis in these areas can be very useful for the practice of health promotion. The last section, 'A sociology of health promotion', takes a somewhat different tack. In this section the sociological method is applied to health promotion itself. This enables a critical analysis to be made of such aspects of health promotion as its norms and values, its ideological underpinning as well as its exhortations to making healthy choices. Finally, this section addresses the question of whether health promotion acts as a form of social regulation.

Sociology is a discipline based on critical analysis. By taking a sociological perspective we are able to contribute to an examination of both the role and efficacy of health promotion. Sociology is able to ask not only What is health promotion? but also, Why does it take the form that it does? Is this the most effective form in its own terms? and, How have we come to define what effective is?

WHAT IS SOCIOLOGY?

Sociology attempts to analyse the world through the processes which constitute it, whether this is on a macro level or on a micro level. The former, which might loosely be called structural sociology, looks at such areas of social organization as the economy, education, religion, and work, and their role in the organization of everyday life. This level of sociology would also examine the workings of the institutions and organizations in which this everyday life takes place: government, industry, schools, families, etc. Sociology would want to know who were felt to be the important people involved. Who benefits from its existence and how? How is it funded? What are its stated aims and objectives? What are its values and assumptions? In short, sociology is asking how society works, at the level of institutions and organizations, and what beliefs and attitudes (ideologies) support or challenge this.

There is another level on which sociology works however, the level of individual behaviour. What do people actually do, and why? How do people make sense of their social world, their family, their schooling, their job? How does this micro level of social behaviour interact with the macro level? The key question is how to integrate the two levels of analysis. What is the relationship between the actions and beliefs of individual people in their daily lives and the structural forces and organizations in which they take place? This is perhaps the heart of sociological enquiry: what is the relationship between individual behaviour (social action) and social structure? Commonly, and too simplistically outlined here, there have been two schools of thought: one that the aggregated actions of individuals are what forms the structures and the other that the structures determine the actions of individuals. More useful, I would suggest, is the notion of a dynamic interaction between individual and social structure with influences and changes moving in both directions.

This has clear relevance for health promotion which is, after all, in the business of facilitating change at the level both of the individual and of the organization or structure.

Once again, sociology's key concepts can be of use. Not only is sociology in the business of analysing social processes but it is also interested in the ways in which society is structured, that is, in describing and analysing the different groups which constitute society. These analyses might include social class, gender, age, race. Of course they are not mutually exclusive categories and the relationships between them are also of interest to sociologists, for example, the interaction between the effects of gender and of age. Finally, how groups and categories come to be defined is of interest to sociologists. What does it tell us about a society where people are conceived of in categories such as age, or class, or gender and not, for example, by eye colour or astrological sign?

Overall then, sociology is concerned with understanding how society is organized and by what processes it is maintained or changed. Historically sociologists have adopted a framework which stresses either conflict or consensus. The conflict theorists roughly follow Marxist or Weberian analyses or some development or integration of the two. These interpretations have in common an analysis of competition between social groups to achieve their own interests; fundamental to them is the inequality between the groups although this is not necessarily thought to be bad. The consensus view acknowledges the plurality of interest groups in society but stresses the harmonious nature of the whole, with each group having its purpose and its place and all functioning in the best interests of society as a whole. This functionalist view is derived from Durkheim's perspective on social organization and one of its notable contemporary exponents has been Talcott Parsons. Interestingly for this discussion, Parsons took health and illness as examples of key factors in the maintenance of social equilibrium. From this, he developed the concept of 'the sick role' (Parsons 1951). In this view, 'illness and illness behaviour' must follow prescribed forms, with the patient, physician, and any others involved having the shared goal of recovery. This functionalist approach to social analysis sees illness as best dysfunctional and at worst deviant (and thus subject to sanctions).

Concepts of *power* are therefore also crucial to a sociological interpretation of the world. More recently macro level theories have been subject to a general critique. Interactionist and ethnomethodological perspectives (Goffman 1959; Garfinkel 1967) draw attention to the importance of the particularity of place. The micro social context in which events take place is integral to their meaning and therefore also to their effect or consequences at both micro and macro levels. Thus, nothing is free of the social context in which it takes place. This kind of theorizing exposed the subjective nature of social life and forced the wider discipline to reconsider its claims to 'scientific objectivity'. The notion of a 'value-free' sociological analysis was revealed as problematic and it became apparent that all theories are generated from within social, political, and economic perspectives. Thus, this theoretical standpoint demands that rigorous analysis acknowledge and articulate these interests and contexts, not proceed as if they do not exist.

It may be more useful to have an analysis which conceptualizes power as a medium rather than an object. In this sense, individuals or groups cannot 'have power' or indeed be rendered powerless. Power can only be exercised, not possessed; it is the medium which exists between social actors, the vehicle through which social relations are expressed.

This more fluid notion of power enables an interpretation of the world which can account for both structural and individual levels of action and the relationship between them (Foucault 1979; Giddens 1979).

These sociological concepts of power, social process, and organization can contribute very usefully to the project of health promotion. I suggest this might take two forms. First, sociological analysis can provide information and understanding which would make health promotion more effective. Second, sociology can offer a critical analysis of health promotion, its theory and its practice. These approaches might be referred to as sociology as applied to health promotion and the sociology of health promotion. The latter parts of this chapter will address these approaches in more depth. First, however, it seems appropriate to consider the relationship between sociology and health.

SOCIOLOGY OF HEALTH AND ILLNESS

Medical dominance

Initially sociology was recruited into the field of health and illness in the service of medicine. Medical education saw the need for its students to understand the relationship between health care and the society in which it takes place. Of prime interest were the concerns of the clinicians. Why, for example, did people consult so often with apparently trivial conditions? What was the relationship between the experience of illness and the decision to seek help? How could doctors ensure compliance on the part of their patients? Indeed, what sort of relationship should a doctor and patient have?

In addition to this, medicine, particularly public health medicine (at that stage in its interim guise as community medicine), needed to know how or indeed *which* social factors contributed to the epidemiology of disease. Data were called for on housing, clients, income, employment, etc.

Thus it is apparent that sociology could assist medicine in its task, both in improving the provision of health care to the individual and in analysing the social origins of disease. In its early days, this was sociology as applied to medicine, with sociology's agenda very much set by the interests of medicine. This approach fits well into the consensus model outlined in this chapter and indeed Parsons was the main exponent of medical sociology during the 1950s.

Medicine as a profession

Early medical sociology developed a related interest in the sociology of the medical profession. Who were doctors? How did they operate as a group?

What were the sociological characteristics of the medical profession and how did they maintain their position? This approach did therefore shift the balance from sociology as applied to medicine to the sociology of medicine, even if this was confined to an analysis of the profession (Freidson 1970; Herzlich 1973). Thus sociology was contributing to medical education and practice, and now was forming a critique of the profession of medicine and the implications of this for the delivery of health care.

Incorporating lay perspectives

The group most obviously missing from medical sociological enquiry were patients. What was their experience of illness, of medicine? How was health maintained and illness dealt with in the lay sphere? What kinds of doctoring did people want? How did they go about getting it?

A cursory foray into this kind of approach immediately calls into question the definitions of health and illness that were in use. Are medical definitions of health and illness those used by a lay population? How might they differ? Indeed, is medicine the sole, even the most important way in which ordinary people deal with their illness? Armstong points out that, until 1954, it was assumed that the experience of symptoms led to a medical consultation:

> The study (Koos 1954) reported that people seemed to experience symptoms much more frequently than their rate of medical consultations would indicate. The researchers were surprised at this because they had assumed, as had medicine for a century and a half, that symptoms as indicators of disease almost invariably led to help seeking behaviour.
>
> (Armstrong 1989: 3)

The significance of this shift in emphasis within medical sociology, from a medical to a lay perspective, was to prompt an intra-disciplinary debate about terminology. 'Medical sociology' evolved into sociology as applied to medicine, and ultimately became the sociology of health and illness (which is now the journal title), which is intended to include all the foregoing aspects whilst not limiting the discipline to a medical agenda (see, for example, Dingwall 1976). This allowed for the discipline to address the relationship between health and other major sociological categories, for example, gender, race, class, age (see examples in Black *et al.* 1984).

This has clear parallels with the disciplinary development of health education and health promotion and their relation to medicine (Rodmell and Watt 1986).

A critique of the medical model

Perhaps most importantly for health promotion, this expansion of sociology's remit has allowed it to produce a critique of the medical model and to undertake the project of understanding how health and illness fit into the experience of everyday life. At a structural level, sociology has criticized medicine as a tool to support capitalist development and exploitation (Navarro 1974; Doyal 1979). Medical dominance in the social world has led to a moral critique (Illich 1976), which charges medicine with creating a dependent 'lay' population which is increasingly reliant on the medical profession. Related to this 'de-skilling' thesis is Illich's charge of iatrogenesis; that is, that, far from healing, the practice of bio-medicine actually creates illness, as for example may result from the risks of surgery, anaesthesia, immunization, or adverse drug reactions. There is also a large critical literature on the role of medicine in mental health (Szasz 1961; Foucault 1967; Sedgwick 1982; Laing and Esterson 1973).

This structural level of critique would also address ways of improving health which take into account the influence of factors traditionally beyond the scope of medicine. These might include employment, family structure, housing, and at a policy level might suggest possible sites of intervention (McKeown 1979; Kennedy 1983; Townsend and Davidson 1982). Understanding how health and illness fit into the experience of everyday life would address lay concepts of health and illness and draw from these lay models of health behaviour which may run counter to or in conjunction with those of scientific medicine. These might include those models/belief systems which are based on class, race, age, or gender experience (Cornwell 1984; Blaxter and Patterson 1982; Dingwall 1976; Thorogood 1990) or which consider systems of health care which exist outside the bio-medical model, that is, alternative or complementary therapies.

Finally, perhaps the field of sociology of health and illness allows a critical perspective on the social role of medicine. This would examine aspects of social life which may be subject to medical regulation. Clearly any claim to sickness ultimately requires medical sanction, e.g. for work or school. But we also see the 'medicalization' of many other areas of life, e.g. pregnancy and birth, alcohol abuse, immigration laws (TB), crime and deviance. There are few areas of social life on which medicine doesn't have an 'expert' opinion, and sociology can offer insights into how and why these processes take place.

Health promotion can therefore clearly benefit from sociology's interest in these areas. What is it that a sociological perspective can add to the theory and practice of health promotion?

SOCIOLOGY AS APPLIED TO HEALTH PROMOTION

Health promotion makes claims to know not only what constitutes healthy behaviour, but also the best way to go about encouraging people to achieve it. For this, health promotion needs an analysis of the different groups which constitute society: men and women; young and old; rich and poor; black and white. It relies on knowledge of these groups' varying beliefs and attitudes, interests, and concerns. Health promotion, then, implicitly depends on sociological categories when pursuing its ends.

If health promotion's project is to address change at an individual or a structural level, it needs to know the 'raw material' it is working with. It needs to know what people mean by health, how they believe it affects their lives, and what they feel they could or should be doing about it, in order to facilitate any effective behaviour change. Sociology's analysis of power is crucial if health promotion is to acknowledge the constraints on, and the potential for, social change. Sociology, then, is vital for providing the theoretical insights into the nature and practice of health promotion.

The contribution that a sociological perspective can make to the discipline of health education and health promotion largely depends on what the aims and goals of health promotion and education are thought to be. Clearly, views on this will vary both within and without the field. However, let us assume here the broad-based, loose definition that health promotion is about increasing people's control over their own health, and that this goal is to be attained by addressing the twin supporting themes or pillars of lifestyle and structuralist approaches (WHO 1984, quoted in this volume p. 7). This definition raises a number of questions, some of which will be addressed in this chapter. It will however serve, I hope, as a description of the discipline broadly acceptable to most interested parties.

Lay beliefs

Beginning from this point, it is clear that sociology can provide insights at a number of levels. First, let us consider the role of lay beliefs. There is much sociological evidence that 'the medical model' of disease causation and illness is not uncritically adopted by the non-professional community. Blaxter and Patterson (1982) for example undertook a three-generational study of health attitudes and behaviours amongst a group of working-class Scottish women. They found a whole range of explanations were employed as to the cause of a disease, including individual susceptibility, infection and environment, familial tendencies, stress, poverty, and others. These explanations were clearly influenced by the social context of these women's lives: their own relative poverty, their often damp housing; their role as daughter, mother, or grandmother; their age; their own interpretations of illness or scientific medical explanations.

Indeed, for this group, the authors conclude, *cause* is the most important aspect. Diagnosis alone is insufficient, what these women wanted to know was *why* they had got it. This is not uncommon: social and medical anthropologists (Helman 1978; Cornwell 1984; Herzlich 1973; Pill and Stott 1982) all point to the need for people to explain illness and disease in terms of their own experiences – why me? why now? (Tuckett 1976). They also acknowledge that these explanations will imply certain actions, whether these be the traditionally prescribed 'doing the month' (Pillsbury 1984) of Chinese post-partum rituals or the commonplace English aphorism 'feed a cold and starve a fever' (Helman 1978). These authors also alert us to the different layers of belief and explanation. What a person may find acceptable as a general explanation of why people get certain forms of disease, may not necessarily be employed as sufficient explanation as to why *they* have got it. Cornwell (1984) distinguishes two levels of account, the public and the private, which characterize this. Thus, other people may have brought it on themselves by neglecting some aspect of approved behaviour, e.g. inadequate hygiene, food, sleep, or excessive smoking, drinking, 'stress', etc. Whereas personally it may be attributed to family disposition, 'bad luck', or environmental influence. Pill and Stott (1982) found a high degree of fatalism about the aetiology of illness amongst their sample of isolated, less well-educated, young, working-class mothers in South Wales. As Stacey explains:

> Ordinary people in other words, develop explanatory theories to account for their material, social and bodily circumstances. These they apply to themselves as individuals, but in developing them they draw on all sorts of knowledge and wisdom, some of it derived from their own experiences, some of it handed on by word of mouth, other parts of it derived from highly trained practitioners. These explanations go beyond common sense in that explanations beyond the immediately obvious are included.
> (Stacey 1988: 142)

Obviously these findings have a number of implications for health promotion's strategies. For example, understanding the complexity of lay beliefs could be important for making health promotion initiatives relevant in their approach to the language and concepts that are used by those they wish to reach. Indeed, health promotion might consider it essential to incorporate the knowledge of these 'lay' attitudes and behaviours into its programme designs and strategies. This would certainly be in keeping with developing a more sophisticated 'lifestyles approach' and would contribute to four of the Ottawa Charter's five principal areas of health promotion action: namely, creating supportive environments, strengthening community action, developing personal skills, and reorientating health services. Of course, 'lay beliefs' do not exist in a vacuum, totally separated from 'professional' explanations. Medical theories and diagnoses are incorporated into everyday explanations of ill health; commonly, for example, germs, bugs, and viruses. Neither is this traffic only in one direction. Doctors are just as likely to employ lay explanations in their diagnoses, perhaps particularly in their dealings with the general public, but also because doctors, too, are 'ordinary people' in some aspects of their lives. As Stacey points out, 'As well as lay concepts being socially situated, so is professional practice socially contextualized such that it is itself influenced by lay modes of conceptualization' (1988: 152). Helman's paper 'Feed a cold, starve a fever' (1978) illustrates this process in a North London general practice.

The study of lay beliefs takes us further than this however. Not only must we recognize the 'cross-over' in concepts and language between the lay theories and the bio-medical ones, but we must also acknowledge a more general acceptance by professional and lay people of the relevance of socio-economic factors. 'Ordinary people' themselves recognize the effect of social structure in defining their scope for action. This leads us to a consideration of the ways in which sociology's analysis of social stratification can contribute to the health promotion project.

Social stratification

A society can be divided up in many ways. The categories chosen, however, will reflect social norms and values. In the contemporary world the most commonly used aspects of social division are class and/or wealth, age, gender, and race or ethnicity. These categories themselves reflect differences in power relations between the groups. It follows therefore that these categories will be relevant to the kinds of health and illness experienced. Much sociology of health and illness has focused on these variables, analysing the multivariate ways socio-economic factors have a bearing on health. It is my intention here, to take each category in turn, considering some examples of the way these aspects of social structure have a bearing on health and illness and therefore indicate the use of this analysis for health promotion.

In the UK the best-known and most comprehensive work on the relationship between social class and health is the report of the Black Committee (DHSS 1980). This report noted that, despite a general improvement over the last century in the population's health, the disparities between classes remained. The Black Report took mortality as the indicator of health and the Registrar General's classification of occupational classes as an indicator of social class. Whilst these are both less than perfect measures in themselves, they work surprisingly well at predicting levels of health. Thus we see continuing inequalities in health between the social classes which show remarkable consistency whether one takes infant mortality, accidental death, incidence of heart disease, or whatever.

Whilst the database and framework for this report are largely epidemiological, the Committee produced four socially based explanations for these
differences. These explanations were:

a   Artefact: this explanation proposed that the results were no more than
    a reflection of the statistical categories chosen.
b   Natural selection: this would explain the preponderance of ill health in
    the lower social classes by suggesting that people with a tendency to ill
    health will be unable to compete favourably in the occupational market
    and thus naturally 'drift down' into the lower social classes.
c   Materialist or structuralist: this proposes that the correlation between
    social class and health is a consequence of the unequal distribution of
    socio-economic factors, such as housing, unemployment, and wealth.
d   Cultural/behavioural: this model attributes health inequalities to the
    'lifestyle' differences between the classes.

The Committee themselves favoured a complex interaction between the latter
two explanations. The far-reaching political implications of these findings
caused the report to be initially suppressed.

There have been many subsequent commentaries on the Black Report,
which both summarize and provide critique of its findings (Hart 1985;
Strong 1990). More recently the work has been updated (Whitehead 1987;
Davey-Smith et al. 1990) to show that these inequalities persist. Indeed
Davey-Smith et al. (1990) maintain that what might have been an effect of
unsophisticated measures of class in the first instance is not only upheld but
accentuated by the use of more complex indicators of social class and health
in their own research ten years later.

Other qualitative studies of health and illness also demonstrate a strong
relationship between material/structural circumstances and the experience
of health and illness. These fieldwork-based sociological studies describe
and analyse this relationship as it occurs in daily life. Some also attempt
to articulate the relationship between socio-economic circumstances and the
products of 'culture', 'lifestyles', or health behaviour (Cornwell 1984; Blaxter
and Patterson 1982).

Once again, it is apparent that sociological analysis has highlighted a key
dilemma for health promotion: the tension between either focusing on
facilitating structural change or concentrating on an individual behavioural
approach is raised again. Clearly the evidence for also taking a structural
level approach for intervention is incontrovertible (Tuckett 1976: Townsend
and Davidson 1982; Davey-Smith et al. 1990) and it is this which has lain
behind the transition of health education into health promotion (Rodmell
and Watt 1986); community medicine into the new public health (Ashton
and Seymour 1988); and the Alma Ata declaration (WHO 1978) into
healthy public policy (amongst other things, see this volume, Chapter
1). This does not by any means imply that the 'lifestyles' approach has

been abandoned but rather that to be effective in increasing individuals' or communities' potential for health the two must be addressed together. Indeed, it must be recognized that the two may be theoretically distinct but are in fact practically inseparable. The nagging question raised here is why it appears that, despite the evidence and the theory, the 'lifestyle' approach still predominates.

It is here that any 'gut feeling' that this is bound to be the case can be given some intellectual credence through sociological analysis. Using the earlier discussion of concepts of power it can be seen that resistance to policies which imply widespread social, political, and economic change is most likely to come from those social groups who have least to gain. Thus, for example, in relation to the debate about the health effects of alcohol, we see the relationship between government and breweries militating in favour of changes in the types of beverage produced and the point or level of advertising but not towards massive increases in taxation or constraints on outlets for purchase or consumption. There are of course many reasons underlying the way policy decisions are made (see Chapter 7 this volume) and, to refer again to the earlier analysis of forms of power, these will be subject to local variation. Thus policy will vary between nations, within them, and of course over time, as the balance of power and resistance shifts between the interested parties. It is, of course, a matter of political perspective as to whether you see this shifting balance as one of consensus or conflict; as between interest groups which are inherently equal or inherently unequal.

This discussion is also equally applicable to the other variables in social stratification mentioned earlier. I will now briefly consider the specific relationship between health and illness and gender.

Gender

There have been many sociological studies which demonstrate the effect of gender. Inequality in almost all areas of social life is structured along gender lines whether this be in employment, education, wealth, family life, or even linguistic use (see, for example, Rowbotham 1974; Stanworth 1983; Barker and Allen 1976; Brannen and Wilson 1986; Spender 1980, amongst many others). This is no less true for health. In the UK the main gender division in relation to health is the difference in morbidity and morality rates. Overall, men have a higher rate of mortality, women a higher rate of morbidity. As Armstrong put it: 'In summary, women get ill but men die' (1989: 46). Sociology's role is to unravel why this should be so. What are the social processes which led to this difference in experience? Or indeed is there a purely biological explanation? Whilst there are *some* diseases which are biologically sex specific (gynaecological ones for instance), it is also true that most diseases affect both sexes. Indeed, as Armstrong (1989) goes on to point out, in other social systems the mortality/morbidity patterns are reversed, so it seems that the explanations are social rather than biological.

Drawing on the literature which documents gender inequalities, sociologists of health have formulated links between the general experience of inequality and the unequal experience of health. Thus again we see class, in terms of employment, housing, poverty, education, all having a bearing, not just on health but differentially on women's and men's health.

Perhaps the single most important factor that distinguishes women's experiences from men's is women's role in the family. This has, of course, been a central tenet of feminist theory (see, for example, Zaretsky 1976; Mitchell and Oakley 1976; Barrett 1980; Delphy 1977; Eisenstein 1979; Millett 1971; Kuhn and Wolpe 1978).

How then does this plethora of research aid the effectiveness of health promotion? It should be clear that understanding and knowledge of differences in gender experiences of health will lead to more specifically focused campaigns. An understanding of the inequalities in gender relations will also lead to a more subtle and effective approach to the structural changes needed to promote health. For example, knowledge of the unequal distribution of resources within families (Brannen and Wilson 1986) would lead healthy public policy initiatives to address levels of child benefit (as it is paid directly to women) rather than family income support (which is not). Initiatives on healthy diet would address (as they have) women's almost total responsibility for the purchase and preparation of the household's food. Indeed, should health promotion, for the benefit of women's health, challenge these accepted social roles?

Given the breadth of the topic, it is of course here possible only to cast a cursory glance at issues of gender and health and I have concentrated mainly on differences in the experience of health and in the responsibility for health within the family. This neglects one large area of health in which gender is highlighted; that is, the provision of health care. Women are the main providers of health care in both the public and the private spheres, as both paid and unpaid carers (Stacey 1988). This too should feature in the setting of health promotion's aims and strategies at both the individual and collective level.

Age

Age is yet another variable which can determine health status and behaviour. It is clearly a target area for health promotion too since different age groups have specific health characteristics. Obviously, the growing proportion of people in society who are over the age of 60 is of particular pertinence to the makers of health and social policy. How this work is done may be influenced by sociological analysis.

Should policy makers, for example, be addressing the more general inequality in the distribution of resources for this age group? Should they be using sociological analysis to examine how this might be an effect of their low status as a social group, or whether their low social status is an effect of their lack of resources? Does health promotion have a role in campaigning not just for policy and lifestyle changes but in the whole social and cultural construction of 'the elderly person'?

The same might be said about other socially constructed 'age groups' such as 'middle-aged men', 'fertile women', 'children', or 'youth'. Indeed each group does have socially specific characteristics which are related to their experience of health and their health behaviour. It follows too that health education and promotion has long since directed its gaze towards influencing the health and behaviours of these groups. What has perhaps not been explicit is the role of sociology in identifying these people as 'social groups' and in analysing their particular relationships to power. This will of course have a strong bearing on their capacity for social action and resistance as both individual actors and as collectivities. See, for example, Oakley (1984) on women and child bearing; Dorn (1983) on youth subcultures as a 'buffer' to alcohol education; Phillipson (1982) on the construction of old age.

Race, religion, culture, and ethnicity

This final category is somewhat harder to define, for the categories themselves are far from fixed or even subject to a general consensus. Nevertheless, one powerful way in which contemporary social inequalities are structured is along lines of 'race'. This is best understood as a political rather than a biological category (IRR 1982a, 1982b, 1985, 1986; Sivanandan 1983; CCCS 1982) in which it is the common experience of racism (as structured oppression) which unites the group. This definition includes aspects of religion, culture, and ethnicity. For example, in the UK currently religious groups such as 'Muslim' and 'Jewish' would be appropriate, but not the Church of England (and note it is not to do with the size of the group in question, but its ideological dominance, or lack of it). Cultural groups such as 'the working class' or 'Northerners' might be considered relatively powerless but not others such as Chelsea fans or claret drinkers. Ethnicity as a concept also depends on an uncritical acceptance of 'common sense'. This renders 'Asian' but not 'American' an 'ethnic group', Irish but not English.

Since, once again, these categories represent inequalities in power they also therefore represent inequalities in health. Although there may be diseases which are more prevalent amongst some race/ethnic/cultural groups than others (e.g. sickle-cell anaemia, tuberculosis, heart disease; see Bhat et al. 1988), these differences, as with gender, may not be fundamentally biological. The higher incidence of tuberculosis amongst 'Asians' in the UK may have more to do with their social conditions as an effect of racism than a biological predisposition. These sociologically defined inequalities can also help explain why some groups have been targeted for health education and promotion intervention rather than others. The consequences of this have however not always been straightforwardly beneficial. It is these 'unintended consequences' of health promotion (itself a debatable phrase) which will be examined in the next section.

This section has addressed the way in which sociological analysis can be used to further the health promotion project. This might be done by 'addressing' aspects of social stratification such as class, gender, age, and race by taking account of the differential nature of power relations between groups, or by explicating the exchange of concepts between 'lay' and 'expert' belief systems. Sociology can make explicit the taken for granted and thereby facilitate more effective targeting of policies and campaigns.

It remains to be asked whether sociology *should* be facilitating this kind of increased effectiveness, this depth of penetration. In whose interests is it? How were these interests defined? How does it fit with the previous analysis of power? The next section moves to a critique of health education promotion.

A SOCIOLOGY OF HEALTH PROMOTION

This approach asks not what sociology can contribute to the increased effectiveness of health promotion, but *what* is the role of health promotion and can it be uncritically regarded as 'good'? Sociological enquiry can reveal the norms and values which underpin health promotion; it might also ask questions about the nature of health promotion as a discourse.

Norms and values

Previously, Tuckett (1976) addressed the choices for health education from a sociological perspective. He distinguished the three main reasons for health education as being a) to act as a branch of preventive medicine, b) to facilitate effective use of health care resources, and c) to provide general education for health. These reasons, he continued, involve health education in choices about ethics and politics and questions of value judgement. They raise questions about what 'healthy' and what 'normal' are.

At this point in the recent history of health education the debate was focused on whether health education could be effective by encouraging individual change *without* demanding any wider social or political change. Tuckett (1976) presented the well-documented and now widely accepted evidence (see this chapter) that health education intervention at a *social* level is likely to be much more effective than simply targeting individual lifestyles and behaviour. Tuckett's argument turned on the point that *all* health education is political (i.e. not to demand a change in the status quo is

itself a political act). If it is accepted that this is the case, then arguing against
health education taking a political role is invalid.

Here then are signs of the first stirrings of the shift to health promotion,
to the goals of Health For All 2000 and healthy public policy which are now
so readily adopted. All intervention for health, must, according to Tuckett:
'Consider and influence relevant social norms and values . . . and health
norms and values do not exist independently of other norms and values in
society' (1976: 60).

Application of this kind of sociological theorizing has led to some
very trenchant critiques of the practice of health education (e.g. Rodmell
and Watt 1986; Farrant and Russell 1986). Take, for example, Pearson's
(1986) excellent exposure of the racist ideologies underpinning many health
education campaigns directed at ethnic minorities. She takes as case studies
the campaigns about surma, rickets, antenatal care, and general dietary
education. These, she reveals, concentrate on 'lifestyle' aspects of 'Asian'
behaviour whilst failing to acknowledge those social structural factors which
might be contributing to the overall health outcomes. For example, the
campaign about lead in eye cosmetics (surma) ignored factors such as the
amount of lead acquired in the blood stream from water pipes in the old
housing available to this group, or indeed from paint or the effect of being
constantly in an inner-city traffic-filled environment. Similarly, rickets has
been eradicated in the white British population by national level policy to
fortify commonly used food items with the necessary vitamin D. In contrast,
the Asian rickets campaign suggested more 'lifestyle' changes: eating more
cornflakes and more margarine and exposing themselves to more sunlight.
The case is similar with the Asian mother and baby campaign, where late
antenatal booking was implicitly assumed to be the problem of the client,
not a consequence of the way the service was delivered.

Ideological underpinnings

Application of the sociological method of critical analysis, however, takes
us further than the individual vs. social structure debate. We reject the
'victim blaming' approach so admirably revealed by a close examination of
the effects of concentrating on 'lifestyles' health education. But the level of
analysis employed by Pearson (1986) allows us to see the *ideologies* which
underpin such strategies. It is not, she says, simply that 'victim blaming' is
wrong; that the 'lifestyles' approach is ineffective; it is that these policies
are racist, depending as they do on a particular socially constructed view
of 'Asian'. This view constructs 'Asians' as a homogeneous group, subject
to a single but all embracing 'culture'. This undifferentiated group is also
constructed as particularly prone to certain diseases as a consequence of their
ethnic origins (which may of course be highly varied). Action to improve
this 'disease proneness' is assumed to be best undertaken by individuals (by

changing their lifestyles) but this is regarded as impossible due to the rigid nature of their all-embracing, but now constructed as conservative, culture. This ideology therefore constructs the notion of an 'Asian culture' which is pathological, and indeed a pathological Asian population. Most revealing of all, however, is that the discourse which underpins this ideology is that of scientific medicine. To be Asian is bad for your health; it is no accident that 'pathological' is the term employed.

This kind of critical analysis shows how important it is, not only to 'consider and influence relevant social norms and values' (Tuckett 1976: 60) with regard to the 'target group' for health education and promotion, but also to examine the social norms and values and the underlying ideologies of those doing the targeting.

This critical approach is apparent in a number of other areas. Hilary Graham, for example, in her work on smoking in pregnancy and amongst mothers of young children (1987) shows how health-promoting strategies recommended by health educators and promoters do not take into account the material realities of these women's lives. It is not simply that they cannot afford the recommendations; indeed, in the case of smoking they may well stand to gain financially. Instead, it is that it simply does not make sense, in the context of their daily routines, to adopt these strategies. As Graham shows, when trapped at home all day with young children and little disposable income, smoking makes sense. You cannot have a physical break from this full-time caring responsibility, you cannot even shut yourself away for half an hour or take a lunch break as another worker would. You must be constantly physically present, alert, and available. Sitting down for ten minutes with a cup of coffee and a cigarette can provide a much needed break to this routine. In addition to which, the costs are low and the calories few.

Making healthy choices

The implications for health education and promotion of this kind of sociological study is that the picture may not be as straightforward as it seems. Definitions of 'healthy' and 'normal' are not fixed. 'Choice' is not equally available to all people and choices are themselves circumscribed by material conditions. As Graham concludes in her earlier work on women's roles as carers:

> From the picture of family health which emerges in this book, routine and not choice is the concept which policy makers and professionals need to confront. For choice occurs within, and is contoured by, the routines of everyday life.
>
> (Graham 1984: 188)

'Choice' is a key concept in health education and promotion and one which bears closer examination. As the example above demonstrates, 'choice' is constructed and constrained by many factors. Kerr and Charles' (1983) work on food and diet within households similarly shows that factors which are equally important for promoting and maintaining family health can sometimes be in opposition to the healthy behaviour promoted by professionals. For example, the key to many 'white British' families' dietary pattern is contained in the socially significant notion of 'a proper dinner'. 'A proper dinner', as Murcott (1983) has shown, is central to women's role of caring for the family. As Graham goes on to summarize:

> A cooked dinner is seen to constitute a proper meal. Correctly served it consists of 'proper' and 'real' vegetables. Sausages and baked beans do not qualify on either score, whilst chops and peas do. The Sunday dinner epitomises proper eating, for both children and adults; in many families it may be the only occasion on which they eat fresh vegetables (Kerr and Charles, 1983: 11). Kerr and Charles noted in their survey of mothers in York that, in eating properly on Sunday, some families found themselves forced to eat badly (in their terms) throughout the week. The cost of meat, in particular, can force families to make cuts in their consumption of other foods, in fruit and fresh vegetables for instance.
>
> (Graham 1984: 132)

The important point here for health promotion is that 'healthy behaviour' is not uncomplicatedly related to material circumstances. It has a symbolic element which can be of overriding importance when determining 'choice'. Sociology's role is to draw attention to this.

A critique of health promotion's strategies

This suggests some attention must be paid to the methods employed by health education/promotion. The simple knowledge–action–behaviour change implicit in many health education campaigns is shown to have, at best, limited success (Tones 1986). Developments in health promotion have suggested that this information-giving approach is a necessary but not a sufficient condition for change. Alongside it should be an 'empowerment' model which emphasizes both 'rationality and free choice' (Tones 1986: 7). This is to be achieved through facilitating decision-making skills and clarification of values and will promote collective social and political action by acknowledging the structural constraints on free choice. A more sophisticated approach to this is the community development model. This acknowledges that 'the community' in question will have pre-existing knowledge and values which will influence the way in which information is received and acted on, choices and decisions made. It recognizes too that these communities might also have something to offer.

The remaining strategy for health promotion/education is the mass market campaign, which is closely related to the first, preventive, information-giving approach. There is no space here for in-depth critique of this model but suffice to say that in its own terms it can never be more than superficial. From a critical perspective it might be asked if advertising can ever be a suitable medium for promoting 'health', which is neither product nor commodity, or for 'selling' a negative message (see, for example, Rhodes and Shaughnessy 1989a).

Thus, health education has been criticized for too narrow an approach, focusing on individual behavioural change in a socio-economic vacuum. Health promotion has acknowledged that good health is not achieved by a series of individually located changes but by situating them in a wider context which both actively promotes and facilitates these choices. What health promotion has perhaps failed to recognize is that 'the healthy choice' is not a unitary concept and that there are many social, cultural, and symbolic meanings which need also to be taken into account.

A recent example of a health promotion campaign which has failed on these grounds is the Health Education Authority response to HIV/AIDS. Many critical works have levied attacks at the 'norms and values' which have been attributed to targeted groups, but also, and perhaps most importantly, to the ideologies and values which have underpinned the campaign but which were not articulated. To quote Simon Watney:

> Hence the intensity of the struggle to define what the syndrome is with the virus being used by all and sundry as a kind of glove puppet from the mouth of which different interest groups speak their values. AIDS, however, has no single truth of its own but becomes a powerful condenser for a great range of social, sexual and psychic anxieties.
>
> (Watney 1988a: 58–9)

Sociologists have highlighted the dilemma facing government-sponsored health education bodies between, on the one hand, the clear need for information on a vital public health issue and, on the other, a political and social reluctance to raise the profile of sex (Wellings 1988; Watney 1988b). The reason for this tension can be revealed as a resistance to undertaking any public education campaign which addressed forms of sexual relationship that might be perceived as undermining 'traditional family values' (Jessopp and Thorogood 1990). What we got was a campaign which gave out muddled messages and it is sociological analyses that can suggest some reasons for this.

Critiques have drawn attention to the racism, homophobia, and eroto-phobia (e.g. Watney 1988b) which have underpinned national HIV/AIDS health education and promotion strategies. The consequences of this, however, are not simply to increase prejudice but to reduce the effectiveness of these measures. The targeting of 'high risk groups' draws attention away from the fact that it is the behaviour, not the group membership, which carries the risk, thereby engendering complacency amongst those whose sexual behaviour is 'risky', but whose group membership identity is not. It also fails to make the information relevant to the lives of the target group.

As Holland *et al.* (1900a, 1990b) make very clear in their work, national health/education campaigns directed at young people have neglected to take gender relations into account. This is crucial since the 'prevailing definition of sexuality can also render girls relatively powerless to define what happens in an individual sexual encounter' (1990a: 8). Young women are encouraged to take responsibility for protected sex whilst no consideration is given to the context of power relations in which their relationships take place. As Holland *et al.* say elsewhere in this paper;

> Government health education policy on the risks facing young women is currently totally uninformed on the social constructions of female sexuality.... Knowledge of young women's sexuality needs to be analysed if health education is to be effective in helping to contain the AIDS epidemic.
>
> (Holland *et al.* 1990a: 3)

Sociological analyses of power and the relationships between individual agency and social structure are therefore vital for making health education and promotion campaigns relevant to the target groups' lived experiences. Sociology is necessary for articulating the framework within which 'choice' can be exercised, and for understanding how adjustments to this framework might be made. In the example of young women's supposed responsibility for safer sex we see not only how socially constructed gender relations act to make girls both responsible and blameworthy but also how the dominant values of male sexuality and patriarchal ideology have underpinned health education and promotion strategies so far. This may render them less effective in achieving behavioural changes but it does serve to reinforce the social, political, and ideological status quo.

Health education and promotion as social regulation

Perhaps sociologists should be asking whether there are consequences of health promotion which lie beyond facilitating healthy behaviour. Does health promotion act as an agent of social regulation? Are 'healthy choices' themselves an expression of prevalent social norms and values?

As we have seen, choice is constructed and constrained by socially organized power relations, which themselves create the routines or 'normal' relations in which 'choice' is exercised. In order to facilitate making the healthy choice, health promotion must take these factors into consideration. We have also seen that there are other discourses, social, cultural, symbolic, which influence decision making.

Health promotion, not surprisingly, supposes making the *healthy* choice to be the most important. It therefore assumes that this is also how any rational person would act. The task for health promotion is then to remove obstacles, both individual and social structural, to this choice. To quote Ashton and Seymour:

> Health Promotion works through effective community action. At the heart of this process are communities having their own power and having control of their own initiatives and activities. . . . Health promotion supports personal and social development through providing information, education for health and helping develop the skills which they need to make healthy choices.

> (Ashton and Seymour 1988: 26)

Although progressive health promotion rhetoric is keen to emphasize the principle of ethical voluntarism (Tones 1986); that is, the freedom to make any choice, it is clear that some choices are assumed better than others. It is further assumed that once in possession of the information, the clarified norms and values, and the decision-making skills, and with socio-cultural barriers removed, any rational person could not help but make the healthy choice. Thus, healthy behaviour is seen to be synonymous with rational behaviour. This discourse of rationality belongs within the medico-scientific paradigm which itself defines health and disease. This focus therefore privileges the healthy choice and obscures decisions made in other discourses. This may be the maintenance of family values and cohesion though the provision of a 'proper dinner' or smoking as a strategy for coping with bringing up small children, or it may be the regulation of safer sex within heterosexual relationships. Indeed we might ask why the discourses of health should be expected to have any prominence in decision making about sex at all. Indeed, it is only in the realm of medicine that 'sex' is considered 'health behaviour' and then it is addressed only in terms of its outcomes, e.g. pregnancy, contraception, abortion, STDs, etc. For most people the role of 'sex' in their everyday lives is not primarily a health concern. More likely to feature are discourses of risk, pleasure, danger, and penetration; and whilst these formulations of experience remain unacknowledged, so the health promotion message will remain ineffective, as the work of Holland *et al.* (1990a, 1990b) and Wilton and Aggleton (1990) in relation to HIV has so clearly shown.

Here then is an inherent tension for health promotion. To acknowledge the possibility of choice within discourses other than health as equally valid would undermine health promotion's claim to scientific rationality. If health promotion were truly to accept all choices as equally valid, the role of *health* promotion would be reduced to promoting access to and decision making about services, and the dominance of the rational, medico-scientific paradigm would be challenged. It would be possible for other social formations to arise, for competing social norms and values to move into ascendance.

At this level, then, health promotion can be conceptualized as a form of social regulation. By allying itself to scientific objectivity, health promotion can continue to promote 'healthy choices' as value free and rational. In doing this it may fail to acknowledge other discourses and simply act to perpetuate existing social relations.

CONCLUSION

This chapter has aimed to outline the broad basis of the sociological method and to consider the contribution this method has made or might make to health promotion. First, it seems that knowledge generated initially through medical sociology and subsequently through the sociology of health and illness can make a valuable contribution by questioning definitions of 'health' and by examining the social role of medicine. Second, we have seen how sociology can be a useful tool for increasing the effectiveness of health promotion. This might be through analysis of social structure, identification of relevant target groups, consideration of the role of lay beliefs, or in weighing up the relevant merits of individual versus structural approaches. Third, we have seen how a sociological perspective can contribute to a critique of health promotion, both in its methods and in its goals and aims.

What, then, can be concluded about the relevance of sociology for health promotion? I would suggest that a strong case can be made for the inclusion of this disciplinary method in the theory and practice of health promotion for several reasons. The contribution of sociology to the analysis of health and illness has been most notably to challenge medical dominance in defining what health and illness/disease are. It has shown us the narrowness of a medical perspective and the need to recognize other notions of health and illness if we are to understand the experience of everyday life. Obviously, for a practice which seeks to promote 'healthy behaviours' amongst a 'lay' population these insights are invaluable.

As the section on sociology as applied to health promotion demonstrates, the use of sociological categories is implicit in the work of health promotion. Acknowledging and articulating this serves to make health promotion more effective in targeting its work. It also serves to alert health promotion's practitioners to the values and assumptions inherent in these categories. This is clearly necessary if the practice is to be responsive to its clients' needs, to be self-aware, self-critical, and accountable.

Finally, because sociology is a discipline based on *critique*, it allows questions to be asked about the nature of health promotion. It can ask questions about the goals and aims of health promotion and examine their consequences in a wider social context. It is not enough for health promoters simply to 'get on with their jobs', they must also be asking themselves those key sociological questions: in whose interests is this? how is power being exercised here? which values are being prioritized? Use of the sociological method can and should contribute to the theoretical and pragmatic decisions regarding the future of the health promotion project.

REFERENCES

Aggleton, P. and Homans, H. (1988) *Social Aspects of AIDS*, London: Falmer.

Armstrong, D. (1989) *An Outline of Sociology as Applied to Medicine*, London: Wright.

Ashton, J. and Seymour, H. (1988) *The New Public Health*, Milton Keynes: Open University Press.

Barker, D. and Allen, S. (eds) (1976) *Dependence and Exploitation in Work and Marriage*, London: Longman.

Barrett, M. (1980) *Women's Oppression Today*, London: Verso.

Bhat, A., Carr-Hill, R., and Ohn, S. (1988) *Britain's Black Population*, Aldershot: Gower.

Black, N., Boswell, D., Grey, A., Murphy, S., and Popany, F. (eds) (1984) *Health and Disease: A Reader*, Milton Keynes: Open University Press.

Blaxter, M. and Patterson, E. with assistance of Sheila Murray (1982) *Mothers and Daughters: A Three-Generational Study of Health Attitudes and Behaviour*, London: Heinemann Educational Books.

Brannen, J. and Wilson, G. (eds) (1986) *Give and Take in Families: Studies in Resource Distribution*, London: Allen Unwin.

CCCS (1982) *The Empire Strikes Back*, London: Hutchinson.

Charles, N. and Kerr, M. (1986) 'Just the way it is: gender and age differences in family food consumption', in Brannen, J. and Wilson, G. (eds) *Give and Take in Families: Studies in Resource Distribution*, London: Allen Unwin.

Cornwell, J. (1984) *Hard Earned Lives*, London: Tavistock.

Davey-Smith, G., Bartley, M., and Blane, D. (1990) 'The black report on socio-economic inequalities in health ten years on', *British Medical Journal* 301 (18–25 August): 373–5.

Delphy, C. (1977) *The Main Enemy*, London: Women's Research and Resources Centre.

DHSS (1980) *Inequalities in Health: The Black Report*, London: HMSO.

Dingwall, R. (1976) *Aspects of Illness*, London: Martin Robertson.

Dorn, N. (1983) *Alcohol, Youth and the State*, Bromley: Croom Helm.

Doyal, L. with Pennell, I. (1979) *The Political Economy of Health*, London: Pluto.

Durkheim, E. (1964) *Rules of Sociological Method*, New York: The Free Press.

Eisenstein, Z. (ed.) (1979) *Capitalist Patriarchy and the Case for Socialist Feminism*, New York: Monthly Review Press.

Farrant, W. and Russell, J. (1986) *The Politics of Health Information*, London: Institute of Education, University of London.

Foucault, M. (1967) *Madness and Civilisation*, London: Tavistock.

——(1979) *Discipline and Punish: The Birth of the Prison*, Harmondsworth: Peregrine.

Freidson, E. (1961) *Patients' Views of Medical Practice: A Study of Subscribers to a Prepaid Medical Plan in the Bronx*, New York: Russell Sage Foundation.

——(1970) *Profession of Medicine: A Study of the Sociology of Applied Medicine*, New York: Dodd, Mead.

Garfinkel, H. (1967) *Studies in Ethnomethodology*, Englewood Cliffs, NJ: Prenctice-Hall.

Giddens, A. (1979) *Central Problems in Social Theory*, London: Macmillan.

Goffman, E. (1959) *The Presentation of Self in Everyday Life*, Garden City: Doubleday.

Graham, H. (1984) *Women, Health and the Family*, Sussex: Wheatsheaf Falmer.

——(1987) 'Women's smoking and family health', *Social Science and Medicine* 1: 47–56.

Hart, N. (1985) *The Sociology of Health and Medicine*, Ormskirk: Causeway.

Helman, C. (1978) 'Feed a cold, starve a fever: folk models of infection in an English suburban community, and their relation to medical treatment', *Culture, Medicine and Psychiatry* 2: 107–37.

Herzlich, C. (1973) *Health and Illness: A Social Psychological Analysis*, London: Academic Press.

Holland, J., Ramazanoglu, C., and Scott, S. (1990a) 'Managing risk and experiencing danger: tensions between government AIDS policy and young a women's sexuality', *Gender and Education*, 2 (2): 193–202.

Holland, J., Ramazanoglu, C., Scott, S., Sharp, S., and Thompson, R. (1990b) 'Don't die of ignorance – I nearly died of embarrassment', paper presented to the fourth Social Aspects of AIDS Conference, London.

Illich, I. (1976) *Limits to Medicine*, London: Marion Boyars.

IRR (1982a) *Roots of Racism*, London: Institute of Race Relations.

——(1982b) *Patterns of Racism*, London: Institute of Race Relations.

——(1985) *How Racism Came to Britain*, London: Institute of Race Relations.

——(1986) *The Fight Against Racism*, London: Institute of Race Relations.

Jessopp, L. and Thorogood, N. (1990) 'No sex please, we're British', *Critical Public Health* 2: 10–15.

Kennedy, I. (1983) *The Unmasking of Medicine*, London: Paladin.

Kerr, M. and Charles, N. (1983) *Attitudes to the Feeding and Nutrition of Young Children: Preliminary Report*, University of York.

Kuhn, A. and Wolpe, A. M. (1978) (eds) *Feminism and Materialism*, London: Routledge & Kegan Paul.

Laing, R. D. and Esterson, A. (1973) *Sanity, Madness and the Family*, Harmondsworth: Penguin.

Maclean, M. (1986) 'Households after divorce: the availability of resources and their impact on children', in S. Brannen and G. Wilson (eds) *Give and Take in Families: Studies in Resource Distribution*, London: Allen & Unwin.

McKeown, T. (1979) *The Role of Medicine*, Oxford: Blackwell.

Millett, K. (1971) *Sexual Politics*, London: Sphere.

Mitchell, J. and Oakley, A. (1976) *The Rights and Wrongs of Women*, Harmondsworth: Penguin.

Murcott, A. (ed.) (1983) *The Sociology of Food and Eating*, Aldershot: Gower.

Navarro, V. (1974) *Medicine under Capitalism*, London: Croom Helm.

Oakley, A. (1984) *The Captured Womb*, Oxford and New York: Blackwell.

Parsons, T. (1951) *The Social System*, New York: The Free Press.

Pearson, M. (1986) 'Racist notions of ethnicity and health', in S. Rodmell and A. Watt (eds) *The Politics of Health Education*, London: Routledge & Kegan Paul.

Phillipson, C. (1982) *Capitalism and the Construction of Old Age*, London: Macmillan.

Pill, R. and Stott, N. C. H. (1982) 'Concepts of illness causation and responsibility: some preliminary data from a sample of working class mothers', *Social Science and Medicine* 16: 43–52.

Pillsbury, B. (1984) 'Doing the month: confinement and convalescence of Chinese women after childbirth', in N. Black *et al.* (eds) *Health and Disease: A Reader*, Milton Keynes: Open University Press.

Rhodes, T. and Shaughnessy, R. (1989a) 'Condom commercial', *New Socialist* June/July 34–5.
——(1989b) 'Compulsory screening', addressing AIDS in Britain 1986–1989 Campaign, 23 January 1989.
Rodmell, S. and Watt, A. (1986) *The Politics of Health Education*, London: Routledge & Kegan Paul.
Rowbotham, S. (1974) *Hidden From History*, London: Pluto.
Sedgwick, P. (1982) *Psychopolitics*, London: Pluto.
Sivanandan, A. (1983) *A Different Hunger*, London: Pluto.
Spender, D. (1980) *Man Made Language*, London: Routledge & Kegan Paul.
Stacey, M. (1988) *The Sociology of Health and Healing*, London: Unwin Hyman.
Stanworth, M. (1983) *Gender and Schooling*, London: Hutchinson.
Strong, P. M. (1990) 'Black on class and mortality: theory, method and history', *Journal of Public Health Medicine* 12(3/4): 168–80.
Szasz, T. (1961) *The Myth of Mental Illness*, New York: Harper & Row.
Thorogood, N. (1990) 'Caribbean home remedies and their importance for black women's health care in Britain', in P. Abbott and G. Payne (eds) *New Directions in Sociology of Health*, London: Falmer.
Tones, B. K. (1986) Health education and the ideology of health promotion: a review of alternative approaches, *Health Education Research* 1: 3–12.
Townsend, P. and Davidson, N. (1982) *Inequalities in Health*, Harmondsworth: Penguin.
Tuckett, D. (1976) *An Introduction to Medical Sociology*, London: Tavistock.
Watney, S. (1988a) 'AIDS, "moral panic" theory and homophobia', in P. Aggleton and H. Homans (eds) *Social Aspects of AIDS*, London: Falmer.
——(1988b) 'Visual AIDS – advertising ignorance', in P. Aggleton and H. Homans (eds) *Social Aspects of AIDS*, London: Falmer.
Wellings, K. (1988) 'Perceptions of risk – media treatments of AIDS', in P. Aggleton and H. Homans (eds) *Social Aspects of AIDS*, London: Falmer.
Whitehead, M. (1987) *The Health Divide: Inequalities in Health in the 80s*, London: HEA.
WHO (1978) *Alma Ata Declaration*, Copenhagen: Regional office for Europe.
Wilton, T. and Aggleton, P. (1990) 'Condoms, coercion and control: heterosexuality and the limits to HIV/AIDS education', paper given at the fourth Social Aspects of AIDS Conference, London.
Zaretsky, E. (1976) *Capitalism, the Family and Personal Life*, London: Pluto.

Chapter 4

The contribution of education to health promotion

Katherine Weare

Education is an older field of study than health promotion or health education. Many of those who are currently working in health education, and some of those who work in health promotion, came to their careers through the study of education, usually in training to be and practising as teachers. Educational theory and practice have shaped health promotion and health education in fundamental ways, and many of the controversies within health promotion have antecedents in educational arguments. This chapter will examine some of the fundamental goals and insights of education, and explore their relationship to health promotion and health education.

This chapter is divided into two parts. The first part explores two fundamental aims of education, which are to increase autonomy and to initiate learners into 'ways of knowing', and examines the relevance of these two aims for health promotion and health education. The second part of the chapter outlines some of the principles of education that facilitate effective teaching and learning, and reviews the extent to which current initiatives in health promotion and health education are working within these principles.

EDUCATION AS THE DEVELOPMENT OF AUTONOMY

What autonomy means

Philosophers of education maintain that the central goal of education is to enable people to be autonomous. To be educated is essentially to be free, in control of one's own life, able to think rationally and logically, and make decisions without coercion or fear (Peters 1966; Dearden *et al.* 1972).

Education has to be distinguished from training, which has been characterized by Seedhouse (1986) as 'encouraging people to acquire a set of pre-set beliefs, habits and values'. Education is not about persuading a person to do what others think they should. Education is for the person educated: it is they who are the 'client', not the teacher, the paymaster, or the employer. Clearly education is not always synonymous with what happens in the educational system, where often the activity could be more accurately described as 'training'.

Education is not just about the freedom of the individual: it inevitably has a social purpose and a social impact. People cannot be autonomous in isolation: their rights and freedoms depend on how those around them behave and what the social structures within which they live allow them to do. Education for autonomy means shaping a society in which it is possible for people to be free, while ensuring that the freedom of one individual or group is not at the expense of others. How to achieve a balance between the freedom of the individual and the rights of others is in practice a thorny problem.

Naturalism: education as 'freedom from'

Within the theory and practice of education there have been many debates about how autonomy should be interpreted in practice. These debates are often fundamentally about whether human nature is intrinsically good, evil, or neutral. Those who believe in natural goodness see all people as having the blueprint for being a decent human being embedded firmly within them at birth. Education for autonomy is a 'freeing from' the forces that warp the otherwise healthy development of the self. This position has been called 'naturalism' and has been enormously influential. Rousseau is usually credited with being one of the first naturalists. He believed that the task of the educator is to 'get back to nature', find out where the student is, and help them to develop their intrinsically good self. Carl Rogers, a modern naturalist, believes we need a 'person-centred education' where people are allowed to be themselves, to be authentic human beings, fully human and fully present in the world (Rogers 1967).

In this century, naturalism has found an expression in the progressive, child-centred movement in education. This movement has interpreted autonomy as the freedom of the learner to discover his or her own truth (Holt 1970); the task of the teacher is to make the space in which this discovery can take place and then interfere as little as possible. At the far end of the spectrum, some educators have suggested that student autonomy should extend to the right to decide whether to attend formal schooling, and the 'free school' movement emerged (Kozol 1972). Others have suggested that society would be better without the restrictive influence of schools at all, and that we need to 'deschool', and indeed deprofessionalize society as a whole (Illich 1973).

The theory of 'education as discovery' had a strong impact on mainstream school education in the 1960s and 1970s. In Britain many primary schools organized their learning as an 'integrated day' and encouraged 'topic work', giving children a good deal of freedom to choose and move between different activities as they wished. Secondary education was not so touched by this approach, but the major curriculum projects and initiatives such as Nuffield Science, the Humanities Curriculum Project (Schools Council 1970) and 'mode three' syllabuses for the Certificate in Secondary Education were essentially about encouraging students to engage in independent enquiry.

Environmentalism: education as 'freedom to'

A less optimistic educational theory maintains that the educator must play a more active and influential role than the discovery approach allows if autonomy is to be realized in practice. This position has no official name: for ease of understanding this chapter will label it 'environmentalism'.

Environmentalists believe that educators need to work with a realistic understanding of what people are like, how they think, learn, change, feel, and behave, and the outside influences that shape them. Even if people are naturally good (and the environmentalists claim there is not much evidence to support this assertion), they can be easily drawn towards evil by their circumstances. Education is not itself indoctrination, but it is up against the indoctrination to which people are subjected and which shapes their beliefs, attitudes, and behaviour in a very profound way. In trying to overcome this indoctrination and help people reject the superstitions, myths, and prejudices with which they have usually been filled by their experience, education must use tactics that are at least as powerful as those used by the forces that spread the propaganda (Rubinstein and Stoneman 1970; Freire 1973; Postman and Weingartner 1971).

If people are to be free from pernicious influences, environmentalists believe, they need more than good intentions: they need the competencies to put intentions into practice. These competencies include the knowledge addressed by the discovery learning approaches, but go further to encompass attitudes and behavioural skills, for example the ability to 'say no' to unwanted pressure. Teaching such competencies involves the educator in organizing the learner's experiences in a very proactive way.

Education for a free and just society

Just as many debates about education and the individual have been centrally concerned with whether people are naturally good or naturally evil, so debates about education and society are often ultimately about the fundamental nature of society. Both naturalists and environmentalists believe that a 'free society' does not mean one in which there is unrestrained competition and 'survival of the fittest': there must be a balance between the freedoms of the individual and the needs of others, so that the strong give support to the weak rather than exploit them. Naturalists believe that a just and fair society will emerge automatically as intrinsically good people, freed from negative influences, negotiate and construct social rules which are self-evidently for the good of all. Environmentalists see this as too optimistic, and maintain that the achievement of a fair society requires active intervention. According to the environmentalists, the task of education is to instil positively the attitudes, values, and skills which are needed for society to be a place in which all can be free, such as tolerance, giving support, and sharing.

Within environmentalism there are also shades of opinion. The more politically radical of the environmentalists suggest that society is essentially a scene of conflict where those in a position of power tend to exploit those not so fortunately placed. They maintain that, in order to avoid the disruption that would occur if the oppressed were aware of their oppression, the truth is obscured and suppressed by a great deal of ideological propaganda spread by, for example, the media and the education system (Bourdieu 1974; Althusser 1966). They regard the naturalist vision of society as a benign place in which equal individuals negotiate their way to consensually agreed solutions as naive, and in some sense as part of the propaganda which keeps an unfair social structure in place. They believe that education should be about 'raising the consciousness' of those at the bottom of the social pile to help them change society (Rubinstein and Stoneman 1970).

The model of 'education as raising political consciousness' achieved considerable status as a theory in the late 1960s and early 1970s through the study of radical social science. The impact of this model on the practice of education was much smaller. It fullest development was in the community education of Paolo Freire in South America (Freire 1973). In Britain and the United states it mostly found an outlet in the classroom practice of individual teachers (Searle 1972; Kozol 1968; Kohl 1971), although the William Tyndale primary school adopted it as school policy until prevented by the famous 'inquiry' (Auld 1976).

Education as empowerment

Since the beginning of the 1980s, the most influential educational initiatives have focused on the individual. The emphasis has been on teaching skills to 'empower' people to take charge of their own lives and get along with other people. Popular examples are the 'Lifeskills' manuals and books produced by the Counselling and Career Development Unit at Leeds University (Hopson and Scally 1981; Hopson and Scally 1979–88) and several initiatives connected with the development of assertiveness (Townsend 1985). Such approaches have been seen as being politically conservative (Rodmell and Watt 1986), but the authors of the 'Lifeskills' programmes contest this most vehemently. They claim that the empowerment of individuals is a necessary precondition of desirable social change, and that unless individuals are skilled at both asserting their own needs and respecting the rights of others then structural change will do nothing to end exploitative relationships but will just put new individuals in positions of power (Hopson and Scally 1981). However, if personal skills are to be translated into social change, overt links need to be made for the learner as to how this is to take place. Such links may be being made elsewhere, but to date they have not yet been included in any published 'Lifeskills' type programme.

Autonomy in practice

So far in this chapter it has been suggested that the key debates of education are concerned with how to create the conditions for the growth of autonomy in the learner and the creation of a free and just society. To gain a sense of perspective on such debates it must be remembered that they are the province of those few people who are concerned with educational theory and the development of progressive initiatives. Such work is almost invariably a long way from the policies of those who shape education and the practice of those on the ground who deliver it. Teaching and learning in schools and in the workplace has not on the whole been centrally concerned with autonomy, at an individual or societal level. Most teaching and learning that takes place in the real world is training.

The social forces that shape educational systems do not tend in the direction of greater autonomy for people, individually or collectively. Those who live in Western democracies tend to be highly critical of the extent to which the education offered by political systems unlike their own can be described as 'indoctrination', but blind to the ways in which their own education system reinforces and reproduces economic and ideological structures. Few are aware that the original force behind the creation of mass education in the nineteenth century was not a philanthropic urge to enlighten and empower. Mass education was created as a tool to form cohesive structures and solve the 'problem of order' that had emerged with the breakdown of traditional social patterns during the Industrial Revolution, and to 'gentle the masses' so that they would accept industrialization and urbanization (Bowles and Gintis 1976). Teaching and learning was then, and still is, largely about acceptance of the rules of others.

In Britain since the beginning of the 1980s even the rhetoric of autonomy has been in decline. The 'right-wing backlash' is calling for a return to traditional didactic methods and a re-emphasis on the learning of facts and teacher-centred formal approaches (Cox 1981). The stated aims of education are increasingly to equip people to fit into the needs of the market-place. Conformity and socially acceptable behaviour rather than autonomy and freedom of thought are the goals (Jones 1989).

Autonomy and health promotion

The dilemmas posed by the principle of autonomy in education are mirrored in health promotion and health education. According to the World Health Organization there is no conflict between the goal of autonomy in education and the goals of health promotion, as the goal of health promotion is to empower people to make their own decisions about health. This aim is reflected in the definition of health promotion offered in the Ottowa Charter: 'health promotion is the process of enabling people to increase control over, and to improve their health' (WHO 1986). The WHO would claim that, in a choice between the goal of autonomy and the goal of good health, the health promoter must choose autonomy. The WHO sees health as 'a resource for everyday life, not the objective of living', and would claim that a state of good physical health which a person had not freely chosen and over which they did not have control could not be described as good health at all in the sense of 'complete physical, social and mental well-being' as the person could not be said to be socially and mentally 'well' if she or he was being coerced.

The language of autonomy and empowerment falls easily from the lips, but the practice is never easy or comfortable. It is even more difficult for most of those involved in health promotion than it is for those involved in education. The logical consequence of accepting autonomy as a goal is to agree that if educated people choose to act in an unhealthy way then, provided it does not impinge on the freedom of others, this must be seen as an acceptable end result of an educational process (Tones 1981). It is usually very hard for those who wish to promote health to feel satisfied with such an outcome. It cuts across the highly normative goals and values of the health-related discipline, such as medicine or nursing, in which health promoters are often trained. In practice health education and health promotion have always trodden an uneasy path between the goals of education and training, between naturalism and environmentalism, and between conservative and radical approaches.

From the mid-1970s, autonomy in some form has been a theoretical aim of almost all of the most influential school and college health education projects. They have all been to some extent concerned with helping people make judgements, choices, and decisions about their health. Up to the mid-1980s many of the major health education projects had the somewhat naturalist approach of aiming to change knowledge and attitudes, in the belief that if people know what is good for them and feel strong enough to take the right decision, then appropriate behaviour will naturally follow. The names of some of the projects reflect this orientation: *Free to Choose* (Teachers' Advisory Council on Alcohol and Drug Education 1983), *Facts and Feelings about Drugs but Decisions About Situations* (Dorn and Norcroft 1982a), *Drinking Choices* (Simnett et al. 1982), and *My Body* (HEC 1983), all have the ring of personal freedom and choice.

Some of the health education projects of the late 1980s have been somewhat more environmentalist, in that they concentrate on teaching behavioural skills as well as knowledge and attitudes, for example *Health Matters* (Beeles 1986) and *Health Skills* (Anderson 1988).

All the major health education projects since the 1970s have been environmentalist in so far as they see the educator as having an active role to play in organizing the conditions of learning and in directing the students to engage in certain activities. They are themselves fairly directive and have emphasized the need for dissemination courses, initiated by the project team, in which practitioners can be introduced to the project's new concepts, methods, and materials. Many projects have not been prepared to release materials to those who have not been on the accompanying course.

The activities offered on courses usually reflect a balance between, on the one hand, the naturalist 'learner-centred' approach of encouraging participation, finding out where people are starting from, negotiating the curriculum, and 'facilitating' the learners' outcomes and, on the other hand, the environmentalist 'teacher-directed' approach of the structured 'workshop', where aims, activities, methods, and time are planned in advance. As a result, the courses often teeter between education and training. (The fact that most of the courses call themselves 'training' is a confusion which we will not allow to hold us up here.)

Courses can be described as education, in other words congruent with the goal of autonomy, when the emphasis is on the process of learning rather than on a prescribed outcome, and when dissension is held to be a valid response. When the goal is that learners leave the course with 'approved' values and behaviours, and the course assessed as having failed when this has not occurred, then the course could more accurately be described as 'training'. Some recent projects are most definitely training, for example, the *Skills for Adolescence* project (Teachers' Advisory Council on Alcohol and Drug Education 1988) which has proved to be highly acceptable in the United States and Europe, under a variety of titles. Its goal is to help young people develop conformist values such as self-help, obedience, politeness, sobriety, and moderation rather than to help them to think for themselves or to challenge the situations in which they find themselves.

Meanwhile, others involved in health education and health promotion have been focusing on different goals. Chapter 1 of this volume has mapped out some of the different models of health promotion that have evolved, including the radical movement that complements the strand of radical environmentalism in education. As we have seen in Chapter 1, this radical movement calls for health education and health promotion to 're-focus upstream' by addressing the social and political causes of ill health rather than focusing on the individual 'lifestyles' that are seen as being the effects of these underlying conditions. It is suggested that health promotion should call attention to social inequalities, unmask the propaganda and vested interest that shapes society's health, mostly for the worse, and empower people to challenge and change the social structure (Mitchell 1984). The World Health Organization's view of what changes are needed to achieve 'health for all by the year 2000' is unequivocally radical, with calls for an increase in community action, the creation of supportive social environments, a reduction in social inequality, and the reorientation of the health services (WHO 1986).

As Chapter 1 suggests, to some extent this radical approach has surfaced in the practice of health promotion. The 'new public health' movement (Ashton and Seymour 1988) in Britain, and the World Health Organization's 'healthy cities' network in Europe are examples of attempts to improve health through changes in social policy. Radical approaches are examined on most of the diploma and master's courses in health education and health promotion (Aggleton et al. 1989) and in the initiatives and projects of the large number of groups and organizations devoted to community development (Martin and McQueen 1989). Within school and college health education, some projects have attempted to 'raise the consciousness' of learners (Dorn and Norcroft 1982b) and include a 'community action' approach (Gray and Hill 1987).

However, much health promotion and health education practice could be justly accused of supporting the status quo by having little social awareness, by attempting to instil socially acceptable behaviour rather than encouraging people to change society, and by 'blaming the victim' for their lack of health (Rodmell and Watt 1986; Dorn 1981). As such it could be seen as reinforcing unhealthy social conditions rather than tackling them.

EDUCATION AS INITIATION INTO 'WAYS OF KNOWING'

Traditionally education has mainly concentrated on cognitive development. The common-sense view is that cognitive development involves examining the world directly with the sense organs and finding out what is the case, or becoming aware of what it is that other people have found out and adding it to one's store of knowledge. Philosophically this view has been developed into the school of thought called realism. It is founded on the assumption that the world is an orderly place, governed by scientific laws of causality which give rise to predictable, verifiable, and repeatable events. Objects are real, exist independently of the knower, and relate to one another in regular and largely quantifiable ways. The task of the scientist is to discover, name, and classify the objects and discover the laws that govern their relationships. The task of the learner is largely to learn the conclusions that others have come to about these objects and their relationships, which involves memorizing facts and applying them in the appropriate situation.

Realism is still the most ubiquitous theory of knowledge and of education. Much of Western natural science until recently has been founded on it; positivist social science and psychology still are. It underlies much traditional school education, especially of a scientific kind, and is strongly reflected in the thinking and planning of Britain's national curriculum. It can be found in a very pure form in most undergraduate medical education in which, despite some bold attempts at innovation, education is still largely concerned with the acquisition of facts about the diagnosis and treatment of disease (Fowler 1987; Weare 1987).

Appealing as this position may be to those who like issues to be straightforward, it does not reflect scientific, psychological, or social reality. Questions of what constitutes truth and knowledge are very problematic. Scientists have for some time cast severe doubt on the common-sense idea of a universe governed by predictable laws, and the recent theory of 'chaos' makes it appear an increasingly untenable position. If such uncertainty surrounds the nature of the objects of the physical world, then those of the social world such as 'good health' are very elusive indeed.

As Chapters 2 and 3 in this volume suggest, psychology and sociology have demonstrated the extent to which the world is a construct of the human mind: what we classify as objects are shaped, and in some ways actively created, by the ways in which our minds perceive them. What we learn from an experience is a feature of what we already know (Ausbel *et al.* 1978), and we learn by adding links to our existing mental framework (Gagné 1965, 1984), assimilating new information into old patterns as far as possible, and accommodating our minds only when the fit becomes too uncomfortable (Piaget and Inhelder 1958). Such a process is paralleled in the development of belief systems in society (Berger and Luckman 1967). Chapter 1 of this volume summarizes the theory of Kuhn (1970), who has demonstrated that what counts as truth, knowledge, and facts is socially generated and historically specific.

If we accept this relativistic perspective, education ceases to be about the learning of facts and becomes instead an initiation into ways of knowing. Cognitive development involves becoming aware that there are many types of truth and that each way of knowing is relative and specific. Even within a so-called 'discipline' there will exist a range of ways of knowing: the rules and understandings of positivist sociology, for example, are very different from those that govern interpretive sociology, and the type of research and practice they generate should not be judged in the same way. Between disciplines the difference may be even more marked: the ways of knowing involved in sociology will often be fundamentally at odds with those of psychology and even more at odds with those of art. Programmes which aim at developing the emotions cannot use the same criteria as those which aim at developing behavioural skills. Education becomes a matter of encouraging learners to be tolerant and respectful of different ways of knowing, and teaching them the skills of operating within a variety of different frameworks.

'Ways of knowing' and health promotion

Health promotion is an eclectic field of study, which draws on many ways of knowing, as this volume shows. Education for health education and health promotion at all levels invariably contains elements of many subjects, particularly biology, the social sciences, philosophy, personal growth, and management studies. Projects and initiatives examine health issues from a variety of different points of view, and call in consultants from different fields.

The theory of health promotion is attempting to face up to the issues raised by its varied parentage and develop a serious intellectual base (Sutherland 1979). However, in many instances, education and practice in health promotion are founded on the simplistic assumption that different ways of knowing can easily complement one another as they are brought to bear on particular health problems to help in their solution. Unfortunately, as we have seen, different ways of knowing are often incompatible with one another, and may well be incompatible with the health promotion activity. The application of the insights of some disciplines, particularly sociology and philosophy, would raise such fundamental questions about the status, nature, and purpose of some health promotion activity that consideration of the issues would prevent the activity ever getting off the ground.

Health promotion as a whole needs to consider the insights of social science and philosophy, integrate them with its practice as well as its theory, make explicit the models, understandings, and values which underlie various types of activity, and recognize that the choices it makes about which approach to use inevitably involve value judgements.

HOW DO WE EDUCATE EFFECTIVELY?

Understand how people learn

If education is about initiating students into different ways of knowing, then understanding the underlying structures, concepts, procedures, and theories of causality that operate within a particular way of knowing is of far greater importance than learning the particular facts that the way of knowing has generated. Facts are needed: without them a way of knowing has no content to process, but the selection of a particular content is to some extent arbitrary as many different types of content can be used to realize the process.

Theories of social change (Tofler 1980) suggest that knowledge is expanding so fast that memorizing enough data for everyday practice is an impossible task, and in any case pointless as much of what is learnt today will be superseded tomorrow. People no longer train for one career: with the changing job market they may tackle several in a lifetime. Data retrieval systems mean that we can call up the facts we need quickly. In this context the most useful skills are being able to solve problems, think rationally and logically, deduce conclusions, generalize, and transfer learning from one context to another (Mayer 1979). Schon (1983) has categorized such learning in the professional context as becoming a 'reflective practitioner'.

Most modern educational theory minimizes the importance of the acquisition of facts and emphasizes the learning of processes (Entwistle and Ramsden 1983; Barrows and Tamblyn 1980; Gagné 1984). Minds are not empty bottles to be filled with facts: what we learn depends on how our minds have been shaped through our previous experience (Coles 1987). Education needs then to be carefully structured to take students through the learning process in an effective and motivating way. Piaget (Piaget and Inhelder 1958) has demonstrated that what is engaging to the learner is the 'nearly new', something with which she or he is largely familiar and therefore can understand, but which contains a note of dissonance which makes it intriguing. Educators need to ensure that the tasks they offer learners follow this principle, and build from the known to the unknown and from the simple to the complex. Bruner (1966) has shown that learning is most effective when it is organized into a 'spiral' in which issues are revisited in increasing depth as time goes on, rather than in a linear series of 'one-off' experiences. Similarly, people learn best when their experiences are brought together and reinforce one another. Effective education does not tackle topics in isolation, but adopts a co-ordinated approach, where the different learning experiences are organized to complement one another by, for example, studying the same issue in different contexts during the same period of time.

Cognitive psychology has shown us that people are more likely to be influenced by their learning if they have had to engage with it actively and make it their own in some way (Bligh 1980). Students need to spend as little time as possible on passive tasks such as reading and listening, and as much as possible in participatory and active learning (Kolb 1984). Behavioural psychology has provided some useful insights into the conditions under which learning most effectively takes place. It is essential, for example, that the cues for learning be clear to the learner, that teaching and learning are based on rewards not punishment, and that feedback is immediate and positive (Bandura 1970).

Health education has led the field of education in finding ways to apply such psychological insights. It has developed a wealth of strategies for accentuating the positive and involving people in their learning, and we have already commented on its emphasis on participatory work in small groups using an active workshop style. Teaching and learning in health education makes use of a very wide range of methods, such as simulations, games, role plays, discussions, and video (Satow and Evans 1982). The 'Health Action Pack' which is the Health Education Authority's major contribution to the health education of 16 to 19-year-olds focuses mainly on the methods that can be used with this age group (Gray and Hill 1987). The principles of co-ordination, integration, and the spiral curriculum have inspired several projects and initiatives, particularly those produced by the University of Southampton (Schools Council Health Education Project 1977, 1982; Schools Health Education Project 1984; Health Education Authority 1989a, 1989b, 1989c; WHO in press). In recent years the notion of integration has become even more powerful with a recognition that the 'taught curriculum' reflects only a small part of the learning: the environment in which learning takes place has to be taken into account in planning health education. The whole institutional context can, if organized effectively, become a health promoting environment (Young and Williams 1989; Scottish Health Education Group 1990; Weare 1989).

Start from where people are developmentally

To be effective, the educational task must be right for the learner. In order to determine what is appropriate, educators need find out where the learner is starting from (Becker 1974).

A strong factor in determining how people respond to their education is their stage of development. People do not develop in a linear way, and the work of child psychologists has shown how the child moves through distinct cognitive stages, each with their own rules and principles of logic and causality (Piaget and Inhelder 1958). 'Stages' are not confined to children: as people age so they change emotionally and attitudinally, and the beliefs, needs, and interests of a person of 16 will be very different from those of the same person at 60.

Abraham Maslow (1971) suggests that human needs exist at various levels. For most people the 'lower' ones must be satisfied before they are able to consider the 'higher' ones. Once a person has the basic necessities to keep alive such as food and water, she or he can move on to more 'long-term' physical needs such as safety and shelter. With physical needs under control, emotional needs can then surface. The most fundamental emotional need is to feel loved and wanted. Not until this is satisfied can a person feel good about themselves and acquire self-esteem. At the highest level are the intellectual needs. These begin with 'self-actualization', which includes personal achievements, creative expression, and self-fulfilment. Ultimately, the most mature people are able to look outside themselves and their immediate relationships and be concerned with wider issues. Altruism and impartial rational understanding are likely to be achieved only if more self-centred needs have already been satisfied.

It is vital that the educator take into account at what level the students are able to operate when planning an educational strategy. The idea of starting where people are has a long and eminent history. Rousseau, with his beliefs about the need to 'educate the child according to his nature', inspired the child-centred education movement that shaped the theory and practice of primary school education in a powerful way. In this century this principle has been applied readily in primary schools and post-compulsory education, but has had little influence in secondary schools (Hargreaves 1972). The recent introduction of the prescriptive national curriculum is likely to make it even less influential, and indeed even primary education is in danger of losing its child-centredness as a result.

The principle of taking into account a person's stage of development is beginning to have an impact on health education. The concept of a 'health career', which provides a description of ways in which an individual's attitudes to a health issue develop over time, has long had a great deal of currency. The *Health for Life Primary School Project* (HEA 1989c) is founded on extensive research into the beliefs young children have about health. The teacher education project *Exploring Health Education* (HEA 1989a, 1989b) recommends strongly that school health educators should attempt to discover where their pupils are, and employ a 'growth and development perspective' in teaching them. Within the national curriculum health education is planned as a 'cross curricula theme' whose content is less prescribed than the core subjects (National Curriculum Council 1990). This may mean that health promotion could act as a small oasis of pupil-centred learning in an otherwise directed environment.

The idea that health promotion must start where people are is far from being universally accepted, and there are still many examples of inappropriate strategies which are at best useless and at worst counterproductive. For example, some initiatives aimed at adolescents (such as the British government's recent anti-heroin campaign) attempt to build their appeal on the attraction of avoiding long-term health problems and minimizing risk. This is likely to misfire badly, as many adolescents are motivated by short-term hedonism, have little concern for their futures, cannot see any point to living beyond 30, and find the idea of risk very seductive. Recognizing the importance of the learner's developmental stage is a strategy that needs to be adopted more widely in health promotion.

Start from where people are emotionally

Emotions play a central role in human life. Whenever we deal with people we are dealing with beings that are fundamentally, some would say primarily, emotional (Freud 1935). The emotional state of the learner will affect how they learn everything, including cognitive and behavioural as well as affective tasks. It is important that educators understand the emotional state of the learner, as it is always a powerful force, blocking or facilitating learning.

The strongest emotions are the ones we have about ourselves. Canfield and Wills (1976) demonstrate the intimate relationship between self-esteem and learning. As Maslow's theory of a hierarchy of need illustrates, unless students feel good about themselves they will find it very difficult to make satisfactory relationships with others, and to learn successfully. Even educators who see themselves as solely concerned with 'higher' intellectual needs, such as the search for truth, morality, and rationality, cannot afford to ignore the more basic emotional and physical needs of students.

According to Coopersmith (1967), self-esteem depends on how we have been treated in the past by other people and the experiences we have had. The amount of respectful, accepting, and concerned treatment that a person has received from those they care about, and the amount of success the person has achieved would seem to be the significant factors.

Educators need to do more than just take the learner's prior emotions into consideration: they need to concern themselves with the emotions that are generated by the educational experience itself. Education invariably affects self-esteem, for good or ill. Although students arrive at school with their self-concepts already moulded by their early experiences, the educators with whom they come into contact have a vital role to play in continuing to shape the images students have of themselves. Educators need to make sure that all students feel respected and liked, and achieve some success. The resultant high levels of self-esteem can partly 'inoculate' students against later threats to their self-regard. Unfortunately some students find that the experience of their education undermines rather than builds their self-esteem.

Emotion is not just something to be taken into account as a factor that helps or hinders cognitive and behavioural learning: many educators see themselves as rightfully concerned with cultivating the affective development of their students, as well as their intellectual and behavioural skills. People can be encouraged to get in touch with their feelings, to be able to identify them, own them, and listen to what they are telling them (Nelson-Jones 1986). Relationship skills are perhaps the most important skills of all in enabling people to lead worthwhile and fulfilling lives: they form a fundamental part of the 'hidden curriculum' within any educational institution, and need to be addressed within the institution as a whole and taught as part of the overt curriculum. Aspey and Roebuck's (1977) research suggests that educators benefit personally and professionally from developing such skills themselves.

Rogers (1983) suggests that the relationship between teacher and taught is an essential determinant of the quality of learning. Good relationships are based on 'respect, empathy and genuineness' which generate an atmosphere of mutual respect and trust that is highly conducive to learning. In developing their relationship skills, learners are most likely to learn by following the example of those they respect and admire. Educators have to try to ensure that their students wish to identify with them, and that their behaviour and attitudes provide positive role models.

Health education has been in the forefront of educational initiatives which both take the learner's emotional state into account and recognize that emotional development is a legitimate goal for education. Many school-based projects have been centrally concerned with developing self-esteem and relationship skills (Schools Council Health Education Project 1977; Health Education Authority 1989c; Clarity Collective 1988) and with the role of the teacher as pastoral tutor and counsellor (Button 1981; Baldwin and Wells 1981). Most in-service education on health education includes work on the affective side of education (Health Education Authority 1989a; Weare in press). In recent years, the focus of some key health education initiatives has moved from the taught curriculum to the total environment of the institution, in which the ethos and the quality of the relationships that exist there are seen as some of the most powerful influences over the health of the people that inhabit it (Young and Williams 1989; Scottish Health Education Group 1990).

Start from where people are socially

The new emphasis on the total learning environment in which health education takes place is encouraging educational institutions to examine their relationships with the surrounding community and is leading to some valuable initiatives (Young and Williams 1989). It reinforces the need for the educator to consider the social context from which students come.

The cultural background of the learner has a profound effect on their response to education and to health promotion messages. The community is not monolithic, but contains many different subcultures based for example on occupational class, geographical origin, ethnicity, religion, and age group. These cultures will each have different meanings, values, and understandings. All groups have their version of rationality and logic and make choices that make sense to them, however irrational or undesirable they may seem to the others (Hymes 1974). For example, Graham (1985) argues that the smoking habits of working-class women are a rational response to the situation they are in, enabling them to cope with what otherwise seem unbearable domestic pressures. Recognizing and respecting the cultural understandings, values, knowledge, and meanings of the learner is vitally important when devising health education and health promotion programmes.

There is copious evidence of the extent to which education can take forms which are culturally inappropriate for pupils from particular social groups, especially those from the working class and ethnic minority groups (Fuchs 1968; Coard 1971). Pupils who see themselves as rejected by their education tend to respond by constructing an identity which is at odds with the values of their teachers, in order to preserve some sense of self-worth (Hargreaves 1967). Willis (1977) points out that many of those students in his study of a secondary school who smoked or abused drugs were underachievers, and argues that 'unhealthy' habits can be partly seen as their way of getting back at an education that they feel does not meet their needs.

Health promoters need to recognize that their own goals and values are culturally specific and may not be appropriate for some groups. Some encouraging examples are emerging of health education and health promotion working with the felt needs of groups rather than imposing their own normative expectations on them (Larbie 1987). Health promoters need to be careful not to alienate those with whom they do not readily identify because they come from different cultural backgrounds to themselves. Otherwise they risk reinforcing the very problems, such as social inequality and lack of access to the health services, that they claim to be tackling.

CONCLUSIONS

There are aspects of educational theory that health education and health promotion have found fairly easy to incorporate into their theory and practice. On the whole these aspects stem from the psychology of education. They include recognizing that effective education involves adopting active and participatory methods and spiral integrated curricula and starting where people are, cognitively, developmentally, and emotionally.

However, if health promotion wishes to work within an educational framework as a whole, it must make more use of the insights of the philosophy and sociology of education. This involves accepting, for example, that education is concerned with the autonomy of the individual and with the creation of a free society, not with persuading people to adopt desirable attitudes and behaviours. The notion of people being free to choose, even if the choice is unhealthy, has to be respected. Education is about initiating people into 'ways of knowing' not teaching them facts, and these ways of knowing may challenge certain approaches to health promotion in fundamental ways. Education means working with people's attitudes and beliefs, some of which will be antithetical to some of the aims of health promotion.

In essence, taking an educational perspective involves examining the taken-for-granted assumptions of the health promoter about what is desirable, right, and proper and being prepared to see these as part of the problem rather than the solution. This is not likely to be easy or comfortable.

REFERENCES

Aggleton, P., Fitz, J., and Whitty, G. (1989) *Professional Development in Health Education: An Evaluation and Programme Review of Activities Supported by the Health Education Authority*, London: Health Education Authority.

Althusser, L. (1966) *For Marx*, Harmondsworth: Penguin.

Anderson, J. (1988) *Health Skills Training Manual*, London: Health Education Authority (restricted to those who attend 'Health Skills' training courses).

Ashton, J. and Seymour, H. (1988) *The New Public Health*, Milton Keynes: Open University Press.

Aspey, D. and Roebuck, F. (1977) *Kids Don't Learn From People They Don't Like*, Massachusetts: Human Resource Development Press.

Auld, R. (1976) *William Tyndale Junior and Infants School Public Inquiry: a Report to the Inner London Education Authority*, London: Inner London Education Authority.

Ausbel, D. P., Novak, J. S., and Hanesian, H. (1978) *Educational Psychology, a Cognitive View*, 2nd edition, New York: Holt, Rinehart & Winston.

Baldwin, J. and Wells, H. (1981) *Active Tutorial Work*, Preston: Blackwell.

Bandura, A. (1970) *Principles of Behaviour Modification*, New York: Holt, Rinehart & Winston.

Barrows, H. S. and Tamblyn, R. M. (1980) *Problem Based Learning*, New York: Springer.

Becker, M. H. (1974) 'The health belief model and personal health behaviour', *Health Education Monographs* 2 (4).

Beeles, C. (1986) *Health Matters*, Cambridge: National Extension College.

Berger, P. L. and Luckman, T. (1967) *The Social Construction of Reality*, Harmondsworth: Penguin.

Bligh, D. (1980) *Methods and Techniques in Post Secondary Education*, Paris: Unesco.

Bourdieu, P. (1974) 'The school as a conservative force', in J. Eggleston (ed.) *Contemporary Research in the Sociology of Education*, London: Methuen.

Bowles, B. and Gintis, H. (1976) *Schooling in Capitalist America*, London: Routledge & Kegan Paul.

Bruner, J. (1960) *The Process of Education*, Cambridge: Harvard University Press.

——(1966) *Towards a Theory of Instruction*, Cambridge: Harvard University Press.

Button, L. (1981) *Group Tutoring for the Form Teacher*, London: Hodder & Stoughton.

Canfield, J. and Wills, H. C. (1976) *100 Ways to Enhance Self Concept in the Classroom*, Englewood Cliffs, NJ: Prentice-Hall.

Clarity Collective (1988) *Taught Not Caught*, Cambridge: Learning Development Aids.

Coard, B. (1971) *How the West Indian Child is Made Educationally Subnormal in the British School System*, London: New Beacon Books.

Coles, C. R. (1987) 'The actual effects of examinations on medical students' learning', *Assessment and Evaluation in Higher Education* 12: 209–19.

Coopersmith, B. (1967) *The Antecedents of Self-Esteem*, New York: W.H. Freeman.

Cox, C. B. (1981) *Education: the Next Decade: a Personal View*, London: Conservative Party Unit.

Dearden, R. F., Hirst, P. H., and Peters, R. S. (1972) *Education and the Development of Reason*, London: Routledge & Kegan Paul.

Dorn, N. (1981) 'A questioning view of health education', in J. Cowley, K. David, and T. Williams (eds) *Health Education in Schools*, 1st edition, London: Harper & Row.

Dorn, N. and Norcroft, B. (1982a) *Facts and Feelings about Drugs but Decisions about Situations*, London: Institute for the Study of Drug Dependence.

——(1982b) *Health Careers Teaching Manual*, London: Institute for the Study of Drug Dependence.

Entwistle, N. J. and Ramsden, P. (1983) *Understanding Students' Learning*, London: Croom Helm.

Fowler, G. (1987) 'The role of the general practitioner in health promotion', in K. Weare (ed.) *Developing Health Promotion in Undergraduate Medical Education*, London: Health Education Authority, pp. 9–16.

Freire, P. (1973) *Education: The Practice of Freedom*, London: Writers & Readers Publishing Co-operative.

Freud, S. (1935) *The Ego and the Id*, London: Hogarth Press.

Fuchs, E. (1968) 'How teachers learn to help pupils fail', in N. Keddie (ed.) (1973) *Tinker-Tailor. . . . the Myth of Cultural Deprivation*, Harmondsworth: Penguin.

Gagné, R.M. (1965) *The Conditions of Learning*, New York: Holt, Rinehart & Winston.

——(1984) 'Learning outcomes and their effects', *American Psychologist*, April: 377–85.

Graham, H. (1985) *Women, Health and the Family*, Brighton: Harvester.

Gray, G. and Hill, F. (1987) *Health Action Pack: Health Education for 16–19s*, Cambridge: National Extension College.

Hargreaves, D. (1967) *Social Relations in the Secondary School*, London: Routledge & Kegan Paul.

——(1972) *Interpersonal Relations and Education*, London: Routledge & Kegan Paul.

Health Education Authority (1989a) *Exploring Health Education: A Growth and Development Perspective*, Basingstoke: Macmillan.

——(1989b) *Exploring Health Education: Material for Teacher Education*, Basingstoke: Macmillan.

——(1989c) *Health For Life: The Health Education Authority Primary School Project*, Walton-on-Thames: Nelson.

Health Education Council (1983) *My Body Project*, London: Heinemann.

Holt, J. (1970) *How Children Learn*, Harmondsworth: Penguin.

Hopson, B. and Scally, M. (1981) *Lifeskills Teaching*, London: McGraw Hill.

——(1979–88) *Lifeskills Teaching Programmes, Manuals 1–4*, Leeds: Lifeskills Associates.

Hymes, D. (ed.) (1974) *Re-inventing Anthropology*, New York: Vintage.

Illich, I. (1973) *Deschooling Society*, New York: Harper & Row.

Jones, K. (1989) *Right Turn: the Conservative Revolution in Education*, London: Hutchinson Radius.

Kohl, H. (1971) *36 Children*, London: Penguin.

Kolb, D. (1984) *Experiential Learning*, Englewood Cliffs,: Prentice-Hall.

Kozol, J. (1968) *Death at an Early Age*, Harmondsworth: Penguin.

——(1972) *Free Schools*, Boston: Houghton Mifflin.

Kuhn, T. S. (1970) *The Structure of Scientific Revolutions*, revised edition, Chicago: University of Chicago Press.

Larbie, J. (1987) *Training in Health and Race*, Cambridge: National Extension College.

Mansfield, K. (1977) *Letters and Journals*, Harmondsworth: Pelican.

Martin, C. J. and McQueen, D. V. (eds) (1989) *Readings for a New Public Health*, Edinburgh: Edinburgh University Press.

Maslow, A. H. (1971) *The Farther Reaches of Human Behaviour*, Harmondsworth: Penguin.

Mayer, R. E. (1979) 'Can advance organizers influence meaningful learning?', *Review of Educational Research* 49: 371–83.

Mitchell, J. (1984) *What's to be Done about Illness and Health?*, Harmondsworth: Penguin.

National Curriculum Council (1990) *Curriculum Guidance 5: Health Education*, York: National Curriculum Council.

Nelson-Jones, R. (1986) *Human Relationship Skills*, Norwich: Cassell.

Newble, D., Entwistle, N. E., Hejka, E. J., Jolley, B., and Whelan, G. (1988) 'Towards the identification of student learning problems: the development of a diagnostic inventory', *Medical Education* 22: 519–26.

Peters, R. S. (1966) *Ethics and Education*, London: Allen & Unwin.

Piaget, J. and Inhelder, B. (1958) *The Growth of Logical Thinking from Childhood to Adolescence*, London: Routledge & Kegan Paul.

Postman, N. and Weingartner, C. (1971) *Education as a Subversive Activity*, Harmondsworth: Penguin.

Rodmell, S. and Watt, A. (eds) (1986) *The Politics of Health Education*, London: Routledge & Kegan Paul.

Rogers, C. (1967) *On Becoming a Person*, New York: Constable.

——(1983) *Freedom to Learn for the 1980's*, Ohio: Charles E. Merril.

Rousseau, J. J. (1965) 'Emile', in W. Boyd (trans.) *The Emile of Jean Jaques Rousseau*, New York: Bureau of Publications, Teachers' College, Columbia University.

Rubinstein, D. and Stoneman, C. (eds) (1970) *Education for Democracy*, Harmondsworth: Penguin.

Satow, A. and Evans, M. (1982) *Working in Groups*, London: Health Education Council.

Schon, D. A. (1983) *The Reflective Practitioner*, New York: Basic Books.

Schools Council (1970) *Humanities Curriculum Project*, London: Heinemann.

Schools Council Health Education Project (1977) *Health Education 5–13*, London: Nelson.

——(1982) *Health Education 13–18*, London: Nelson.

Schools Health Education Project (1984) *Developing Health Education, A Coordinator's Guide*, London: Nelson.

Scottish Health Education Group (1990) *Promoting Good Health: Proposals for Action in Schools*, Edinburgh: Scottish Health Education Group.

Searle, C. (1972) *Classrooms of Resistance*, London: Writers & Readers' Publishing Co-operative.

Seedhouse, D. (1986) *Health, the Foundations of Achievement*, Chichester: Wiley.

Simnett, I., Wright, L., and Evans, M. (1982) *Drinking Choices*, London: Health Education Authority.

Sutherland, I. (ed.) (1979) *Health Education: Perspectives and Choices*, London: Allen & Unwin.

Teachers' Advisory Council on Alcohol and Drug Education (1983) *Free To Choose: An Approach To Drug Education*, Manchester: Teachers' Advisory Council on Alcohol and Drug Education.

——(1988) *Skills For Adolescence*, Manchester: Teachers' Advisory Council on Alcohol and Drug Education.

Tofler, A. (1980) *The Third Wave*, London: Pan.

Tones, K. (1981) 'Affective education and health', in J. Cowley, K. David and T. Williams (eds) *Health Education in Schools*, 1st edition, London: Harper & Row.

——(1987) 'Health Promotion, affective education and the personal-social development of young people', in K. David and T. Williams, *Health Education in Schools*, 2nd edition, London: Harper & Row.

Townsend, A. (1985) *Assertion Training*, London: Family Planning Association.

Weare, K. (1987) 'Developing health promotion in undergraduate medical education: what is happening in our medical schools at present?', in K. Weare (ed.) *Developing Health Promotion in Undergraduate Medical Education*, London: Health Education Authority, pp. 43–4.

——(1989) 'Health promotion in medical schools: some suggestions for action', in

K. Weare and P. Kelly (eds) *Health Education in Medical Education: A Summary of a World Health Organization Consultation held at the University of Perugia*, Southampton: School of Education, University of Southampton, pp. 6–22.
——(in press) 'Relationships, mental health and assertiveness', in World Health Organization *Promoting the Health of Young People in Europe: A Training Manual*, Edinburgh: Scottish Health Education Group.
Willis, P. (1977) *Learning to Labour*, Aldershot: Gower.
WHO (1986) *Ottowa Charter for health promotion*, Geneva: World Health Organization.
——(in press) *Promoting the Health of Young People in Europe: A Training Manual*, Edinburgh: Scottish Health Education Group.
Young, I. and Williams, T. (1989) *The Healthy School*, Edinburgh: Scottish Health Education Group.

Chapter 5

Epidemiology and health promotion

A common understanding

Andrew Tannahill

INTRODUCTION

Epidemiology is widely recognized as an important scientific foundation for health promotion. This chapter addresses the important questions 'What has epidemiology contributed to health promotion?' and 'How might health promotion be better served by epidemiology?'. Broadly speaking, two interrelated problem areas are encountered: these concern, respectively, the way in which epidemiology is currently brought to bear on health promotion and, more fundamentally, the way in which the term 'epidemiology' is commonly interpreted.

WHAT IS EPIDEMIOLOGY?

Many definitions of epidemiology exist. Most are along the lines of the following, which is commonly used.

> Epidemiology [is] the study of the distribution and determinants of disease in human populations.
>
> (Barker and Rose 1984: v)

The contributions to health promotion of epidemiology *thus defined* will now be considered. Basic principles of epidemiological investigation will be described, since understanding of the 'whats' of the role of epidemiology in health promotion is best built on knowledge of the 'hows'. Moreover, it is intended that the account will help 'non-epidemiologists' to interpret epidemiological reports and data, and to work profitably with colleagues whose principal expertise (and socialization) lies in epidemiology. Interested readers may wish to supplement the account given here by turning to one or more of the numerous specialist textbooks covering the subject at various levels of complexity (Friedman 1987; Lilienfeld and Lilienfeld 1980; Mausner and Kramer 1985). In so doing, however, they should beware of the existence of considerable variation in the use of common terms and the attendant scope for confusion. This semantic muddle is particularly regrettable in a discipline whose practitioners pride themselves on the 'hardness' of their methodologies and data.

CONTRIBUTIONS TO HEALTH PROMOTION

These may be considered under headings derived from the above definition: distribution of disease and determinants of disease.

Distribution of disease

The study of the distribution of disease – *descriptive* epidemiology – is central to public health. Its relevance to health promotion lies in its being an essential first step in the prevention of ill health. Descriptive epidemiology, as the name suggests, describes aspects of the burden of disease in communities. These aspects are:

1 the *amount* of given diseases, in terms of deaths occurring over a certain period of time (mortality), cases arising in a particular population over a defined time (incidence), or cases existing in a population at a point of time or over a defined time period (point and period prevalence, respectively); and

2 the manner in which particular diseases are distributed according to characteristics of *time, person,* and *place*.

Much of this work may be done using routinely collected data. Mortality data relate to causes of death, and are obtained from death certificates. Morbidity data are concerned with non-fatal disease events, and are obtained from a wide range of sources, including hospital discharge returns, sickness absence certificates, infectious disease notifications, cancer registrations, general practice records, and the national General Household Survey (which collects medical, social, and other information from a random sample of the population of the United Kingdom).

In many instances, however, the information required is unobtainable through routine channels, and special studies are required. These typically take the form of a *cross-sectional study*, in which the situation in a population at or over a given time is studied, usually through investigating a carefully selected representative sample of the population of interest.

Amount of disease

Routine mortality statistics show, for instance, that the major causes of death in Scotland (as in the United Kingdom as a whole) are coronary heart disease (CHD), cancers, and cerebrovascular disease: in 1988, these conditions accounted for 17,963, 14,720, and 8,150 deaths, respectively, representing 29 per cent, 23.8 per cent, and 13.2 per cent of deaths in Scotland in that year

(Registrar General Scotland 1989). Crude figures of this sort are clearly of value to those concerned with the promotion of health, in that they help build up a picture of the burden of serious ill health in a population.

For any given disease, whether we are dealing with mortality, incidence, or prevalence, it is necessary to relate the number of occurrences of interest to the number in the particular population who are at risk of contributing to these occurrences, and to a specified time scale. In other words, we must calculate a *rate* of occurrence. This is done by dividing the number of occurrences of interest in a specified time (or, in the case of point prevalence, at a particular point in time) by the population at risk. A *crude* rate relates to a total population at risk, for example the total population of Scotland in relation to CHD, or the total female population in connection with cancer of the cervix. Thus it can be calculated using appropriate population estimates that in Scotland, in 1988, the crude mortality rate for CHD was 352.6 per 100,000 population and that for cervical cancer was 7.3 per 100,000 women.

As seen below, however, proper comparisons, over time or between populations, require manipulations of such crude figures, to allow for differences in population structure which may make comparison of crude data invalid.

Distribution by time

The scrutiny of routine data, or the repeated or ongoing execution of special studies, over time allows us to identify and describe time trends for particular diseases. Three basic types of time trend are described (Farmer and Miller 1983: 7).

1 *Epidemic* An epidemic is a temporary increase in the incidence of a disease in a population. Influenza is the classic epidemic disease, with a tendency to relatively short-lived upsurges of incidence of various sizes in and around winter. The 'temporary' may, however, refer to a longer time period, hence present-day references to epidemics of coronary heart disease (see below) and the acquired immune deficiency syndrome (AIDS).

2 *Periodic* This refers to the pattern of more or less regular changes in incidence. For example, whooping cough tends to peak every three years or so.

3 *Secular* Secular, or long-term, trends refer to non-periodic changes in disease statistics over a number of years. For example, tuberculosis mortality has declined markedly, and fairly steadily, since the middle of the nineteenth century. On the other hand, mortality from lung cancer in the UK has grown enormously in the twentieth century. So too has coronary heart disease mortality, although this has shown a decline in recent years (albeit less marked than in the United States and Australia) (British Cardiac Society 1987).

Comparison of disease rates over time requires special manipulations of the crude data to make allowance for possible effects of changes in population structure, notably in relation to age and sex. This is, of course, because most diseases show a predilection for particular age groups, and there are many differences in disease experience between the genders. Thus, a comparison of two crude rates at different times, especially many years apart, may be rendered invalid through the later population's containing a larger proportion of old people or women. The process of *standardization* can correct for age and sex differences simultaneously. Alternatively, separate age-standardized rates for males and females can be calculated.

An important method of standardization involves calculation of the standardized mortality ratio (SMR). This permits comparison between a number of populations by the calculation of a single figure for each population, derived using a reference population. A single SMR can be obtained which makes allowance for differences in age and sex structure between populations. Once again, however, separate figures are often calculated for males and females. Suppose we want to compare male mortality from CHD in Scotland with that in the UK as a whole. The UK male population in this instance is the reference population. Taking the Scottish male population, broken down by age group, we multiply the number of individuals in each age band by the mortality rate in the corresponding age band of the whole UK population (*age-specific* rate). Thus we obtain the number of deaths in each age class which would be expected if Scotland had the same mortality experience as the UK as a whole. The total number of expected deaths for the overall male population of Scotland is then derived simply by adding up the calculated numbers for all the age bands. The SMR is finally arrived at by dividing the observed male CHD deaths (those which actually occurred in the Scottish male population) by the total expected deaths and multiplying by 100.

A population with an SMR of 100 has the same overall mortality experience as the reference population. An SMR >100 indicates a surplus of deaths: a value of, say, 120 represents an excess of mortality of 20 per cent over that which would have occurred had the population experienced the same age-specific mortality as the reference population. An SMR of <100 implies a relatively favourable experience: an SMR of 85, for example, indicates a 15 per cent shortfall of deaths in comparison with the expectation based on the reference population.

SMRs can be calculated for a number of populations, allowing comparison not only with a reference population but with each other. International 'league tables' can be constructed, for example. Moreover, sub-national comparisons may be made: mortality in various cities can be compared, as indeed can the experiences of various districts within cities. Thus, taking the whole of Scotland as the reference population, the SMR for lung cancer in the Greater Glasgow area for the years 1975–88 was 136. For districts within that area, again taking the Scottish population as the standard, the all-causes SMR ranged from around 60 to over 120 (Greater Glasgow Health Board 1990).

The calculation and comparison of SMRs are of benefit to health promotion in quantifying and ranking disease problems, and in identifying places with particularly pressing needs for prevention or other forms of action.

Distribution by person

Characteristics of person which affect the likelihood of occurrence of particular diseases include age, sex, ethnicity, occupation, socio-economic status, marital status, and aspects of lifestyle (such as smoking). Disease rates may be calculated for subsets of the population thus distinguished: for example, we may calculate age-specific mortality rates for accidents (or particular types of accidents), this again helping us to identify priorities for preventive action.

Distribution by place

International, regional, and small area (for example postcode sectors) comparisons of disease distribution may be made. Once more, standardization is required to allow for important differences in population structure.

Determinants of disease

Description of the distribution of disease may throw up some clues as to aetiology, that is to say the causal origins of disease. In other words, descriptive studies may *generate* hypotheses of causation. For instance, a cross-sectional study may show that certain types of respiratory disease are commoner in smokers, leading to the hypothesis that smoking causes these diseases.

Cross-sectional studies may also be used for more advanced exploration into the origins of disease. For example, one such study investigated the prevalence of self-reported symptoms of chronic bronchitis in relation to age, smoking status, and place of residence (characterized as having high or low levels of atmospheric pollution) (Lambert and Reid 1970). Independent associations between the disease (chronic bronchitis) and the suspected risk factors (increasing age, smoking, and atmospheric pollution) were found, but it seemed that in the absence of smoking atmospheric pollution had a relatively small impact.

In general, however, the *testing* of a causal hypothesis requires more sophisticated studies. These may be classified, in order of increasing complexity, as *analytic* (*case-control* and *cohort*) studies and *intervention* studies. Cohort studies will be described first.

Cohort studies

In its simplest form, a cohort study involves recruiting a study population (cohort) free of the disease of interest, categorizing the subjects according to the presence/absence or level of exposure to a suspected risk factor (or risk factors), and following them up over a period of time to see if they develop the disease under investigation. The strength of association between a given risk factor and the disease in question may, in the case of a risk factor classed as present or absent, be calculated by the formula:

$$\text{Relative risk} \quad = \quad \frac{\text{incidence rate in exposed}}{\text{incidence rate in non-exposed}}$$

For a graded risk (such as blood pressure or blood cholesterol level), a separate relative risk may be calculated for a number of classes of risk (for example, diastolic blood pressure 90–99 mmHg, 100–109 mmHg, etc., taking <90mmHg to signify 'non-exposure').

A relative risk of 1 implies an absence of association. Statistical tests are applied to indicate the probability or confidence that the relative risk value truly differs from unity. Subject to such testing, the higher the relative risk, the greater the strength of (positive) association, while a relative risk of less than 1 represents a negative association, suggestive of a protective effect.

It should be noted that positive association, even with a statistically significant and high relative risk, does not necessarily indicate causation. Strength of association, as measured by the relative risk, is only one of a number of factors to be considered in assessing the likelihood that an association is causal (Bradford Hill 1977: 288).

Possibly the most famous cohort study of all time is that concerning smoking and mortality among British doctors, carried out by Doll and Hill (1964). The study involved sending a questionnaire on smoking behaviour to all doctors on the British Medical Register, and following the cohort up for subsequent death. Association between smoking and several causes of death were found. Most notable was the marked association with lung cancer, which, in males, showed a virtually linear relationship between age-standardized mortality rate and number of cigarettes smoked per day.

In terms of health promotion 'message', this study provided evidence that, on a number of preventive grounds, it is advisable not to smoke – or at least not to start. What about people who already smoke? Would they be likely to attain preventive benefits from stopping? A follow-up component of Doll and Hill's classic study offered such hope: analysis of questionnaires enquiring into changes in smoking status demonstrated that the likelihood of dying from lung cancer fell with time after smoking cessation.

The above example dealt with a single risk factor. However, a single cohort study can collect information simultaneously on a number of risk factors. Sophisticated methods of multivariate analysis can then be used to estimate the independent associations of the various risk factors with a particular disease from a morass of potentially interacting risk factors.

The teasing out of the roles of multiple, interacting risk factors is of particular relevance in relation to CHD. Cohort studies such as the Framingham Study (Dawber 1980) have provided much information on risk factors for CHD, their interrelationships, and their relative weights. The most consistently strong independent associations have been found for age, male gender, blood pressure, cigarette smoking, and blood cholesterol level. Combinations of risk factors mark especially high risks.

So far, we have confined our consideration of analysis to relative risk. Cohort studies yield further measures which are of value to health promotion.

1 *Attributable risk* is the incidence of a given disease in the group exposed to a particular risk factor *minus* that in the non-exposed group. This quantifies the hazards, in probability terms, of being exposed to the risk factor and, conversely, the benefits which accrue to an individual from not being exposed (provided, of course, that status as regards that particular risk factor is the only important difference between the groups).

   For example, the attributable risk for cigarette smoking in relation to lung cancer mortality was found in one study to be 169 per 100,000 per year (188 *minus* 19 per 100,000 per year) (Hammond 1966). Provided that the groups of smokers and non-smokers studied did not differ from each other in relation to any other relevant risk factor, this suggests that a person may avoid an excess risk of 169 per 100,000 per year by not smoking (or, more precisely, by never starting to smoke, since the data do not by themselves indicate reversibility of risk).

2 *Population attributable risk per cent* may be calculated in a number of ways, depending on the data available. Broadly speaking, it takes into account, whether directly or indirectly, how commonplace a risk factor is in the population, and is a measure of the percentage of a disease's incidence which may be ascribed to a particular risk factor. It is therefore a guide to the potential benefits to the population of elimination of a particular risk factor. Thus, for instance, it has been estimated that some 30 per cent of all cancers may be attributed to tobacco (Doll and Peto 1981).

Cohort studies are not undertaken lightly. In general they are unsuitable for rare diseases (due to the lack of events of interest), and, even in the case of relatively common diseases, they tend to require a large study population and a long period of follow-up, and accordingly to be expensive. Cohort studies, therefore, should in the main be reserved for the testing of clearly defined hypotheses.

Case-control studies

This type of analytic study often provides evidence which is further explored through cohort studies. On the whole, case-control studies require fewer study subjects and consume less time than cohort studies. Moreover, they are suitable for the study of rare diseases.

A case-control study starts with an identified group of people with the disease of interest – the *cases*, and a suitable comparison group without the disease – the *controls*. The control group has to be 'matched' to the cases in certain important respects (see Barker and Rose 1984: 84).

Cases and controls are then categorized according to the presence/absence (or level) of past exposure to the risk factor(s) of interest. This will often involve enquiry about the past (for example, history of alcohol consumption), giving rise to the possibility of poor or selective recall, which may bias the results. Moreover, the possibility that the factor under study (for example, diet, weight) has been affected by the onset of the disease in question (for example, peptic ulcer, bowel cancer) has to be borne in mind.

Clearly, if there is a positive association between a risk factor and disease, then a higher proportion of cases than controls would be expected to fall into the 'exposed' category.

Unlike cohort studies, case-control studies do not yield incidence rates. Accordingly, relative risks cannot be calculated directly. However, relative risk may generally be estimated with an acceptable degree of precision, by calculating the so-called *odds ratio* from case-control study data.

Just as a number of relative risks may be calculated for a graded risk in a cohort study, so may odds ratios be calculated for various levels of exposure: biological gradients (close response relationships) may thus be identified.

An example of a case-control study of recent relevance to health promotion is that carried out by Winn *et al.* (1981), which showed an association between the practice of snuff-dipping (which involves placing a wad of tobacco, either loose or in a teabag-like sachet, between cheek and gum) and cancer of the mouth. This study has helped secure regulatory action against snuff-dipping products in the United Kingdom and elsewhere.

Experimental studies

Experimental evidence is the benchmark for judging whether an association is causal, and thus for directing preventive efforts. Whereas the types of study described so far involve merely looking at natural phenomena in populations (and are thus collectively known as *observational studies*), experimental studies into causality entail some sort of direct manipulation of the situation by the researchers (and are consequently often referred to as *intervention studies*).

An intervention study involves assessing the effect (in terms of occurrence of the disease in question) of:

1 administering a suspected causal factor (this approach, for obvious reasons, being confined by and large to animal experiments);
2 removing a suspected causal factor (for example, eliminating a suspected industrial hazard from an industrial environment); or
3 employing an agent or device which protects against a suspected causal factor (for instance, using protective clothing as a barrier to a suspected occupational factor).

The distinction between intervention studies (designed to test causal hypotheses) and *preventive trials* (aimed at evaluating the efficacy and safety of particular preventive packages) is blurred in practice. In an ideal world, descriptive, analytic, and intervention studies would establish causal factors. Preventive trials would then help decide how best to combat the identified factors. In reality, however, trials are used not only to assess the impact on risk factors but also to gauge outcome in terms of disease onset or mortality: in other words, to judge causality.

It is helpful to explore the contributions of experimental studies to health promotion using CHD as an illustration. Not only do studies in this area abound, but the wide variation in interpretations of the resulting data clearly demonstrates that the contribution of epidemiology to health promotion is far from straightforward. Also, of course, this disease topic is of particular relevance to health promotion in the developed world, not only by virtue of its place at the top of the mortality league table, but also because the risk factors concerned have been implicated in the aetiology of numerous other diseases and amount to a substantial proportion of the lifestyle components on which health promotion focuses.

The identification of CHD risk factors through observational studies was referred to above. These findings have formed the basis of a broad consensus on action required to prevent the disease. What have experimental studies added to the situation? So far, for reasons which will now be explored, the short answer to this question has to be confusion.

A number of experimental studies in CHD prevention, some centred on people identified as being at 'high risk' and others involving a more or less 'mass' approach, have been reviewed by various commentators (Anonymous 1982; Oliver 1983; Shaper 1987; McCormick and Skrabanek 1988; Shea and Basch 1990). Only two examples will be looked at here, to give a flavour of the polarization of interpretations of major studies.

The World Health Organization (WHO) European Collaborative Trial of Multifactorial Prevention of Coronary Heart Disease involved 60,881 men aged between 40 and 59, working in eighty factories in Belgium, Italy, Poland, and the UK. Half of them received advice on diet, smoking, weight, blood pressure, and exercise (WHO European Collaborative Group 1986).

One commentary on this study discarded it as showing 'no difference in coronary heart disease mortality ... between the control group and the intervention group' (McCormick and Skrabanek 1988). This judgment overlooks important variations between the trial centres. In the Belgian component of the trial, there was a significantly lower total incidence of CHD in those given health education than in the comparison group. Differences of a similar nature, but not statistically significant, were found in Italy and Poland (where statistical significance would be more difficult to reach due to the small number of participant factories and the low population incidence of CHD, respectively). The results of the trial as a whole were weakened considerably by the lack of a positive result (in terms of changes in both risk factors and incidence) in the large UK centre. It could well be that the UK intervention was somehow less suitable or satisfactory than that in other centres.

It will have been noted that the above dismissive critique focused only on CHD mortality, whereas, in Belgium at any rate, beneficial effects of education on the total incidence of CHD were found. Clearly health promotion is concerned with morbidity as well as mortality, and in any case benefits in relation to morbidity might reasonably be expected to precede a reduction in mortality.

It is important to recognize also that the success or failure of health promotion in the prevention of CHD cannot be judged entirely on the basis of an intervention of fairly traditional health education confined to middle-aged men. This brings us to a very different kind of study from the above. The North Karelia Project in Finland followed community pressure for action against CHD. It was set up as a comprehensive, community-based programme, involving health education, specific preventive services, and health protection policies: in other words, action was taken in all spheres of health promotion (Tannahill 1985; Downie et al. 1990: 57). Trends in CHD risk factors and mortality were compared with a neighbouring province and with the rest of Finland (Puska et al. 1983, 1985; Salonen et al. 1983; Shea and Basch 1990; Tuomilehto et al. 1986).

Again controversy reigns in the interpretation of the study's findings. It has been widely accepted that the project led to reductions in CHD risk factors, arguably beyond North Karelia, due to 'leakage' of interest and action (thus, it is said, 'diluting' the impact in North Karelia specifically). However, the commonly propounded conclusion that the interventions in North Karelia reduced CHD mortality in the province has been disputed (McCormick and Skrabanek 1988). Indeed, one of the principal investigators stated that the project 'should not be considered as evidence either for or against the aetiological role of the three coronary risk factors [serum cholesterol level, blood pressure, and smoking]' (Salonen 1987). Returning to a point made above, the project was not in fact designed to test causal hypotheses (in other words, it was not an intervention study proper but rather a non-randomized trial). Scepticism over such studies often distils into a fundamental questioning of the risk factors identified through observational studies. It should, however, be noted that the European Collaborative Trial showed that benefit in terms of CHD reduction was significantly related to the extent of risk factor change.

At this stage of the discussion, it is helpful to move away from specifics, to draw together some very basic points of central importance in appraising critiques of experimental studies concerned with CHD prevention.

1   The lack of unequivocal evidence that preventive intervention reduces CHD mortality does not warrant the conclusion that such interventions have been shown to be useless.
2   Critiques have centred on mortality among the under-65s (in the interests of validity of death certification), whereas, given the age distribution of death from CHD, most of the impact in absolute terms would be to be found in the older age groups (Gunning-Schepers et al. 1989).
3   There is a tendency for commentators to focus on mortality, thus overlooking ignoring beneficial effects on CHD morbidity.
4   The beneficial effects of risk factor change on other diseases (such as smoking on lung cancer, blood pressure on strokes, and obesity on osteoarthrosis and disability) must be taken into consideration. (This points to the absurdity of treating CHD in isolation from other health problems, a point which is explored further below.)
5   Favourable effects of lifestyle change on *positive health* – for example of taking up exercise on well-being and fitness – tend to be ignored by the nihilist camp.

These and the preceding arguments serve as reminders that we must appraise *all* the available evidence, rather than latching uncritically on to debunking critiques. While it is vital to encourage reflective practice, we must resist the unhelpful temptation to caricature challenges to accepted doctrines and dogmas as a nihilistic battle-cry to be taken up as an alternative to addressing the implications for established practices posed by health promotion. Passive acceptance of negative arguments, or the mere succumbing to the created climate of uncertainty and inconsistency, militates against professional and public action towards health promotion.

In short, it would be wrong to convert the much-publicized criticisms of population-based preventive strategies into paralysis. An adequate consensus as to modifiable risk factors remains: we must continue in our search for the best means of altering risk status in the population, and in so doing, we must set our efforts in the broader context of the prevention of other diseases and the enhancement of positive health. These last two themes are of importance to further discussions in this chapter.

Summary of contributions of epidemiology to health promotion

We have seen that epidemiology, as defined at the beginning of this chapter, has an important role in identifying and quantifying ill health problems in communities, in assessing the means of and scope for prevention, and in evaluating preventive interventions.

As we have begun to see in the preceding section, however, the application of epidemiology to health promotion has not been without its difficulties. The problem areas will now be examined, starting with shortcomings arising from the way in which epidemiology is brought to bear on health promotion.

PROBLEM AREAS TO DATE

Unsound programme planning

Epidemiology is generally accepted as a primary feeder discipline for health promotion. In fact it is viewed by many as *the* primary discipline. This is manifest in a widespread tendency to have epidemiology 'drive the system'. That is to say, not only does epidemiology set the health promotion agenda – through identifying and quantifying causes of morbidity and mortality and elucidating foci for prevention – but the resultant catalogue of categories of ill health and risk factors is directly translated into 'health promotion' programmes (figure 5.1).

The end-product is a series, indeed a hotch-potch, of disease- and risk factor-based initiatives. For example, a health authority may devise a CHD prevention programme, a smoking programme, a cancer programme, an alcohol programme, a drugs programme, a human immunodeficiency virus/acquired immune deficiency syndrome (HIV/AIDS) programme, and so on. It is obvious that there are overlaps between such programmes. For example, smoking is associated with CHD and cancers, and tobacco is a drug of addiction; HIV infection is related to illicit drug use and, through effects of intoxication on sexual behaviour, to alcohol use; furthermore, there are common links in the origins of most unhealthful aspects of lifestyle – including factors such as socio-economic disadvantage, unhealthful peer pressure, and the power of vested interests.

Despite these overlaps, the individual programmes commonly proceed in relative, or even absolute, isolation. This lack of co-ordination brings the potential – often realized – for duplication and inconsistency of health education 'messages', which in turn is likely to breed public confusion and rejection.

Furthermore, necessary efforts to secure programmes' permeation of

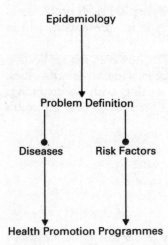

Figure 5.1   Epidemiology driving the health promotion system

whole communities is thwarted at grass-roots level by the inherent unco-ordinated nature of the approach. Important 'gatekeepers' to the community – headteachers, employers, and so on – are likely to be frustrated and irritated by a disjointed stream of requests to take action on this, that, and the other. Even if programmes *are* established in key parts of the community, they will tend to be piecemeal and (as described above) to involve wasteful, and potentially damaging, duplication. These problems and others are discussed more fully elsewhere (Tannahill 1990).

A neglect of methodological issues

The above approach to programme development carries with it important problems regarding methodology. In short, the question of 'how to' is lost in consideration of '*what* to'. Plans become a list of diseases and risk factors to be addressed, often translated into targets for achievement (Tannahill 1987).

Largely implicitly, programmes thus defined rely heavily on outmoded models of health *education*. The assumption is that if people are told what is good – and bad – for them, then healthful attitudes and behaviour will follow in a neat sequence. The consequence of this gross oversimplification (Tannahill and Robertson 1986) is excessive dependence on 'campaigns' and the giving of information and advice, at the expense of notions such as skills development, enabling, and empowerment. This is state of the *ark* practice, not state of the *art*.

An over-emphasis on individual behaviour

Epidemiology-driven health promotion places an onus on the individual member of the public to take responsibility for his or her health, without properly addressing ways of 'making healthy choices easier choices'. Health-related behaviour is largely viewed *in vacuo*, isolated from its social context, and there is a tendency to neglect essential regulatory measures which protect health.

These undesirable features are reinforced by narrow approaches to risk appraisal. For example, CHD has been linked to aspects of lifestyle, including diet and smoking. At the same time, despite frequently being referred to as a 'disease of affluence', it has been shown (Townsend *et al.* 1988) to be associated in the developed world with low socio-economic status. The common response to the latter observation is to point to social class differences in the lifestyle factors, and to return the focus to changing individual behaviour – persuading people not to smoke, and so on – as distinct from the more challenging question of how the broad environment might be changed: individuals are expected somehow to shrug off powerful anti-health pressures in their everyday lives and 'do the right things'. A further problem is that the gradient of CHD across employment groups can, in any case, only partly be explained by orthodox risk factors (Marmot *et al.* 1984).

A narrow view of outcomes

An over-reliance on epidemiology in developing health promotion programmes manifests itself also in the definition of desirable outcomes. These tend to relate to disease incidence rates, mortality rates, risk factor prevalences, and uptake rates for specific preventive services. The contribution of other disciplines towards outcome definition is underplayed. Measures of educational outcome, for example, may be viewed (and indeed played down) as *process* measures.

The narrow outcome focus runs the risk of failing to detect human problems in the operation of preventive programmes. For instance, all-out efforts may be made to pass people through health check programmes, with both eyes firmly fixed on considerations such as uptake and pick-up rates, to the neglect of important matters such as necessary support for risk reduction and potential psychological ill effects of screening.

This brings us to the question of how health is envisaged in current epidemiological practice. So far, we have focused on problems relating largely to how epidemiology is used. It is time to look at those which spring directly from how the term 'epidemiology' is interpreted.

An incomplete view of health

It will be recalled that the definition of epidemiology presented at the beginning of the chapter referred exclusively to disease. Epidemiology seen in this light concerns itself with 'objective' measures of diagnosed disease. The inherent view of ill health is incomplete, in that it overlooks important *subjective* aspects. This may be seen in relation to the above brief discussion of health check outcomes: assessment of psychological ill effects requires the investigation of clients' own feelings and experiences.

Moreover, epidemiology as defined so far is deficient in its neglect of the *positive* dimension of health (which embraces well-being and fitness: Downie *et al.* 1990: 23).

A notable consequence of this incomplete view of health has been the almost exclusive concern with *prevention* in the foregoing account. Indeed health promotion in practice is often reduced to a repackaging of preventive medicine. This is well seen, for example, in many examples of 'health promotion' in general medical practice, and of health authority plans for 'health promotion'. Moreover, as indicated above, the ignoring of positive health is a major weakness in nihilist health promotion writings based on the results of experimental studies.

The case for ensuring an emphasis on positive health in health promotion rests on a number of arguments.

1　Most fundamentally, 'health promotion' which is concerned only with a part of health is obviously a misnomer. This begs the question: what *is* health? A whole series of books could be, and indeed have been, written in response to this question (see Seedhouse 1986; Aggleton 1990). Only a brief analysis of some of the critical issues is possible here.

The classic WHO (1946) definition of health – as a state of complete physical, mental, and social well-being, and not merely the absence of disease or infirmity – is a useful starting point for such a discussion. While this definition is open to valid criticism by dint of its Utopian nature, it is surely of value in embracing the sorts of things which people conceptualize as being part of health. It reminds us that health is not merely to do with the physical – there are important mental and social facets – and that it has a positive dimension.

How does the positive dimension (represented by well-being in the WHO definition) relate to the negative dimension (ill health)? This relationship has generally been represented as a single continuum, with positive at one pole and negative at the other. As pointed out by Downie *et al.* (1990: 20), such a portrayal overlooks the fact that ill health and positive health are by no means invariably inversely related to each other: it is quite possible for someone with a serious disease to have a higher level of well-being or fitness than someone who has a 'clean bill of health' from a clinical point of view. Herein lies a vital lesson for health promotion: successful prevention cannot be relied upon to maximize positive health. This is well illustrated by the extreme image of a society which has taken prevention well and truly to heart, and is accordingly remarkably free of ill health, but which is so concerned with risk reduction that its quality of life is seriously impaired.

Health promotion, then, must surely be aimed at achieving a balance between positive health and ill health, as well as between physical, mental, and social aspects of health.

2 A question of ethic arises from the points made above. Surely it is *unethical* for those involved with health promotion to peddle a pale imitation of the real thing?

Personal experience of a teaching session with clinical medical students provides a suitable illustration. On being asked to define health, one of the students suggested 'the absence of clinical signs'. This met with the approval of his colleagues. However, in an ensuing participatory exercise on perceptions of personal health, consideration of matters of illness and disease was conspicuous by its absence: the students were very clearly concerned with issues of mental and social well-being, physical fitness, and self-concept and self-esteem. They were faced, then, with the dilemma of strait-jacketing patients into a narrow 'medical' view of health while couching their own health in much more positive ways. They could offer no defence for this.

3 It is commonly said that a positive focus is more motivational in terms of encouraging the adoption of a healthful way of life. In strictly academic terms the case for accepting this is commonly overstated. However, there are common-sense reasons for giving credence to the argument. Why should people give up pleasurable (if unhealthful) practices or adopt unattractive (albeit healthful) ones *now* for the sake of some possible – but by no means certain – preventive benefit in the future? This question is particularly pressing in relation to disadvantaged people for whom unhealthful practices, such as smoking or misusing alcohol or other drugs, may be the main pleasures in – and only escape from – an otherwise miserable existence; and for whom the future is neither worthy of investment nor amenable to personal influence. It is also especially relevant to young people, insulated by time from pressing awareness of their own mortality.

4 Also of relevance to the question of motivation is the matter of lay perspectives of health, in which the positive dimension figures prominently. It is clearly important for those who seek to promote health to be operating on a basis with which the public may identify.

5 It is widely accepted that a cornerstone of health promotion is *empowerment*. As well as contributing to this process through informing people and securing environments conducive to health, health promotion can

foster attributes which help individuals and communities to become more empowered. These attributes, including a high level of self-esteem and a set of lifeskills, may be seen as components of well-being: nurturing them, therefore, is part of the process of enhancing positive health.

THE WAY AHEAD

An epidemiology of health

Attention has been drawn to the fact that at present epidemiology is on the whole taken to be concerned with disease, and that this focus is too narrow for effective and ethically acceptable health promotion. Even leaving aside consideration of the impact of epidemiology on health promotion, it is reasonable to suggest that epidemiology should focus on health more fully. After all, although the oldest use of the term appears to have been in connection with epidemics (*Oxford English Dictionary*), the word is derived from the Greek *epi* and *dēmos* and thus means literally 'study on the people', not study of diseases of the people.

The idea of the epidemiology of health was actively endorsed as long ago as the early 1950s, when a book of that title was published in the United States by the New York Academy of Medicine, following a health education conference (Galdston 1953). Galdston referred to the epidemiology of health as 'new', but argued that in actuality it was older than that of disease, and that it was based on an older science – physiology rather than pathology. The book spoke of 'holism', and of an ecological approach, notions which one might have thought of as more modern. A British study of the height, weight, and general condition of two groups of boys was cited as an example of the epidemiology of health, on the grounds that this was a study of the state of health rather than disease. The following definition of the epidemiology of health was presented:

> a discipline, rooted in physiology and trussed by mathematics, whereby essential information on the state of health is to be gained, this information serving to inspire and direct action to maintain and advance the health of the people.

> (Galdston 1953: 6)

Galdston warned that the 'new' epidemiology must not be thought of as 'merely the mirror side of the epidemiology of disease', emphasizing, as has been stressed in this chapter, that health is not the same as the absence of disease.

The epidemiology of health must augment a concern with aetiology and pathogenesis by incorporating methods of enquiry into what it is that enables people to attain and maintain good health in the face of all manner of environmental insults. Kelly (1989) highlighted the need for research focused in this way. Referring to the work of Antonovsky (1987), he advocated the application of a 'salutogenic approach', based on the premise that 'misery, pain, illness and pathology is the normal lot of the human being'. The critical question, he argued, is

> how it is that certain individuals and certain groups, certain households and certain societies are better able to withstand the endemic pathological onslaught of lousy social conditions, of noxious environmental hazards, of self-destructive behaviour, or of micro-organisms, while others are not.
>
> (Kelly 1989)

Pulling together key points made in this chapter, there is a need for epidemiology to focus on the distribution and determinants of good health as well as bad. Just as health embraces the subjective as well as the objective, the positive as well as the negative, the physiological as well as the pathological, then so too must the epidemiology of health.

To what extent is such a vision of epidemiology a reality? This question can be answered to a great extent by reference to the prevailing notion of epidemiology which has shaped this chapter. Although some definitions of the term incorporate the word 'health' (Last 1988: 42; Richards and Baker 1988), and despite periodic 'reinventions' of an epidemiology of health (see Brown 1985, for example), in practice the disease model still dominates.

The picture is not, however, wholly bleak. Conventional, 'objective' measures of ill health have come to be supplemented by well-validated indicators such as the Nottingham Health Profile (Hunt *et al.* 1986), which allows for an assessment of health status based on subjective judgements. In addition to standard epidemiological studies, it has become commonplace for researchers and even health authorities to undertake studies of health-related beliefs, attitudes, and behaviours in defined populations, these representing an extension of the cross-sectional study beyond its traditional territories (see, for example, Butler 1987; Health Promotion Research Trust 1987; Dumfries and Galloway Health Board 1990). The expanded health database provided by such innovations is of value in providing further insights into influences on health, and a population profile of health status and health-related knowledge, attitudes and behaviour, through which health promotion challenges may be identified and progress monitored.

Moreover, much work of the sort described in the New York Academy of Medicine book referred to above has been, and is being, conducted in the name of social sciences or even social epidemiology. Somehow such studies appear to be cut off from 'mainstream' – that is, medical – epidemiology. Such longitudinal studies (for example, the West of Scotland Twenty-07 study: Mcintyre *et al.* 1987) are essentially cohort studies in which subjective and objective assessments of positive health and ill health may be made, and through which determinants of good health and poor health may be explored.

There is a pressing need for the various strands identified here to be pulled together into a unified epidemiology of health. This is not a bid for further territorial expansion by 'medical epidemiology': it is a call for, as it were, a broad church of epidemiology presided over by leaders of many different denominations, in which the importance of lay preachers is recognized.

An integrated base for health promotion

Having made a case for adopting a view of epidemiology broader than that which currently dominates, we need to consider how this expanded discipline should be applied to health promotion.

Criticism was made above of the tendency for epidemiology to drive the system, in the sense that problems identified by the epidemiology of disease come to be translated directly into corresponding programmes of action (Figure 5.1). It was pointed out that this is both philosophically and logistically unsound. As the chapter developed, issues of multi-disciplinary teamwork and sensitivity to lay perceptions and perspectives were raised. Health promotion must involve a partnership between various professionals, many agencies, and the community itself. Health promotion planning, implementation, and evaluation need to be based on an epidemiology of health (itself reflecting such partnership) integrated with other sciences which have a bearing on methodology (Figure 5.2). This is consistent with the argument, made in the introduction to this book, that collaboration in practice must be matched by collaboration in theory.

The necessary coalition of disciplines must be firmly founded on an awareness of each other's perspectives and expertise, and cemented by the mutual respect which is, eventually, born of proper teamwork. This is a vital challenge in these heady days of the renaissance of public health and advocacy of multi-disciplinary, multi-agency institutes of public health. Not least it is a challenge for epidemiologists.

SUMMARY

Epidemiology, as commonly defined, provides important inputs to health promotion, namely: knowledge of the scale and distribution of important disease; an understanding of causal mechanisms, and thus of the potential for prevention; and methodologies for evaluating preventive initiatives.

Major problems arise from the inappropriate application of epidemiology to health promotion: epidemiological evidence on diseases and risk factors tends to be translated directly into health promotion programmes, to the neglect of methodological issues. This problem is compounded by the narrow – disease – focus of mainstream epidemiology, and by its emphasis on 'objective' measures.

There is a pressing need for an 'epidemiology of health', which draws on medical and social epidemiology, and on new methods as well as old.

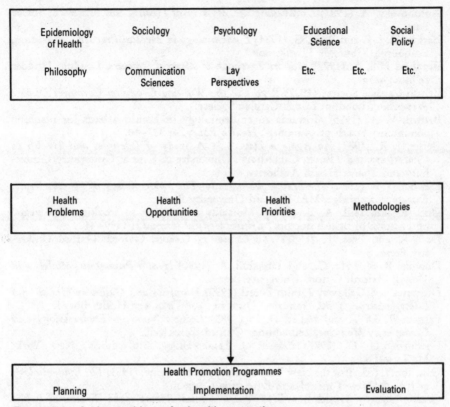

Figure 5.2   An integral base for health promotion

This broader-based epidemiology must recognize positive health together with ill health; it must use subjective measures alongside the objective; it must investigate the distribution and determinants of good health as well as bad; it must seek to identify not only health problems, but also health opportunities; it must be concerned not just with pathological mechanisms, but with physiology; and its view of health determinants must be holistic, so that health-related behaviour is properly viewed in its broad environmental context.

This epidemiology of health must then come to form, with other relevant bodies of knowledge, an integrated, multi-disciplinary base on which health promotion may be planned, practised, and evaluated.

REFERENCES

Aggleton, P. (1990) *Health*, London: Routledge.
Anonymous (1982) 'Trials of coronary heart disease prevention', Editorial, *Lancet* 2: 803–4.

Antonovsky, A. (1987) *Unravelling the Mystery of Health*, San Francisco: Jossey Bass.

Barker, D. J. P. and Rose, G. (1984) *Epidemiology in Medical Practice*, 3rd edition, Edinburgh: Churchill Livingstone.

Bradford Hill, A. (1977) *A Short Textbook of Medical Statistics*, London: Hodder & Stoughton.

British Cardiac Society (1987) *Report of the Working Group on Coronary Disease Prevention*, London: British Cardiac Society.

Brown, V. A. (1985) 'Towards an epidemiology of health: a basis for planning community health programmes', *Health Policy*, 4: 331–40.

Butler, J. R. (1987) *An Apple a Day . . . ? A Study of Lifestyles and Health in Canterbury and Thanet*, Canterbury: University of Kent at Canterbury/Canterbury and Thanet Health Authority.

Dawber, T. R. (1980) *The Framingham Study: The Epidemiology of Atherosclerotic Disease*, Cambridge, MA: Harvard University Press.

Doll, R. and Hill, A. B. (1964) 'Mortality in relation to smoking: ten years' observation of British doctors', *British Medical Journal* i: 1399–410.

Doll, R. and Peto, R. (1981) *The Causes of Cancer*, Oxford: Oxford University Press.

Downie, R. S., Fyfe, C., and Tannahill, A. (1990) *Health Promotion. Models and Values*, Oxford: Oxford University Press.

Dumfries and Galloway Health Board (1990) *Dumfries and Galloway Health and Lifestyle Survey 1990*, Dumfries: Dumfries and Galloway Health Board.

Farmer, R. D. T. and Miller, D. L. (1983) *Lecture Notes on Epidemiology and Community Medicine*, 2nd edition: Oxford: Blackwell.

Friedman, G. D. (1987) *Primer of Epidemiology*, 3rd edition, New York: McGraw-Hill.

Galdston, I. (ed.) (for the New York Academy of Medicine) (1953) *The Epidemiology of Health*, New York: Health Education Council.

Greater Glasgow Health Board (1990) *The Annual Report of the Director of Public Health 1989*, Glasgow: Greater Glasgow Health Board.

Gunning-Schepers, L. J., Barendregt, J. J., and van der Maas, P. J. (1989) 'Population interventions reassessed', *Lancet* i: 479–81.

Hammond, E. C. (1966) 'Smoking in relation to death rates of one million men and women', in W. Haenszel (ed.) *Epidemiological Approaches to the Study of Cancer and Other Chronic Diseases*, National Cancer Institute Monograph 19, US Department of Health, Education and Welfare.

Health Promotion Research Trust (1987) *The Health and Lifestyle Survey*, London: Health Promotion Research Trust.

Hunt, S. M., McEwen, J., and McKenna, S. P. (1986) *Measuring Health Status*, London: Croom Helm.

Kelly, M. (1989) 'Some problems in health promotion research', *Health Promotion* 4: 317–30.

Lambert, P. M. and Reid, D. D. (1970) 'Smoking, air pollution, and bronchitis in Britain', *Lancet* i: 853–7.

Last, J. M. (ed.) (1988) *A Dictionary of Epidemiology*, 2nd edition, New York: Oxford University Press.

Lilienfeld, A. M. and Lilienfeld, D. E. (1980) *Foundations of Epidemiology*, 2nd edition, New York: Oxford University Press.

McCormick, J. and Skrabanek, P. (1988) 'Coronary heart disease is not preventable by population interventions', *Lancet* ii: 839–41.

Mcintyre, S. *et al.* (1989) 'The West of Scotland Twenty-07 study: health in the community', in C. Martin and D. McQueen (eds) *Readings for a New Public Health*, Edinburgh: Edinburgh University Press.

Marmot, M. G., Shipley, M. J., and Rose, G. (1984) 'Inequalities in death – specific explanations of a general pattern?', *Lancet* i: 1003–6.

Mausner, J. S. and Kramer, S. (1985) *Mausner and Bahn. Epidemiology – An Introductory Text*, 2nd edition, Philadelphia: Saunders.

Oliver, M. F. (1983) 'Should we not forget about mass control of coronary risk factors?', *Lancet* ii: 37–8.

Puska, P. *et al.* (1983) 'Change in risk factors for coronary heart disease during 10 years of a community intervention programme (North Karelia project)', *British Medical Journal* 287: 1840–4.

——(1985) 'The community-based strategy to prevent coronary heart disease: conclusions from the ten years of the North Karelia project', *Annual Review of Public Health* 6: 147–93.

Registrar General Scotland (1989) *Annual Report 1988*, Edinburgh: HMSO.

Richards, I. D. G. and Baker, M. R. (1988) *The Epidemiology and Prevention of Important Diseases*, Edinburgh: Churchill Livingstone.

Salonen, J. T. (1987) 'Did the North Karelia project reduce coronary mortality?', *Lancet* ii: 269.

——*et al.* (1983) 'Decline in mortality from coronary heart disease in Finland from 1969 to 1979', *British Medical Journal* 286: 1857–60.

Seedhouse, D. (1986) *Health: The Foundations for Achievement*, Chichester: Wiley.

Shaper, A. G. (1987) 'Epidemiology and prevention of ischaemic heart disease', *Current Opinion in Cardiology* 2: 571–85.

Shea, S. and Basch, C. E. (1990) 'A review of five major community-based cardiovascular disease prevention programmes. Part I: Rationale, design, and theoretical framework', *American Journal of Health Promotion* 4: 203–13.

Tannahill, A. (1985) 'What is health promotion?', *Health Education Journal* 44: 167–8.

——(1987) 'Regional health promotion planning and monitoring', *Health Education Journal* 46: 125–7.

——(1990) 'Health education and health promotion: planning for the 1990s', *Health Education Journal* 49: 194–8.

Tannahill, A. and Robertson, G. (1986) 'Health education in medical education: collaboration, not competition', *Medical Teacher* 8: 165–70.

Townsend, P., Davidson, N., and Whitehead, M. (1988) *Inequalities in Health*, Harmondsworth: Penguin.

Tuomilehto, J. *et al.* (1986) 'Decline in cardiovascular mortality in North Karelia and other parts of Finland', *British Medical Journal* 293: 1068–71

Winn, D. M. *et al.* (1981) 'Snuff dipping and oral cancer amongst women in the Southern United States', *New England Journal of Medicine* 304: 745–9.

WHO (1946) *Constitution*, New York: WHO.

WHO European Collaborative Group (1986) 'European trial of multifactorial prevention of coronary heart disease: final report on the 6-year results', *Lancet* i: 869–72.

Part II

Chapter 6

Using economics in health promotion

David Cohen

INTRODUCTION

A belief that health promotion will reduce health care costs has led many to see health promotion as a way of saving money, and economics as the discipline to highlight where these savings can be made. This shows a lack of understanding both of the objectives of health promotion and of the role that economics can play in the pursuit of those objectives.

While it is possible that money may be saved through health promotion, this is not its primary objective. If saving money were the sole objective, then any health gains which could be achieved only at positive cost would not be pursued. Since virtually all programmes of treatment and cure achieve health gains at a positive cost, such a restriction on health promotion would be absurd.

Economics provides the framework for considering how efficiently health promotion achieves its objectives and how health promotion resources can be used most cost effectively. Economics also provides an analysis of health-promoting behaviour and of the incentives that exist to prevent ill health or to engage in activities that damage health. Such appraisal and analysis can produce essential information for devising, planning, implementing, and evaluating health promotion programmes.

To appreciate how economics can play these roles, this chapter begins by explaining basic economic principles, highlighting the fact that economics is first and foremost a way of thinking. This is followed by a discussion of how economics offers an alternative analysis of health-affecting behaviour and the implications this can have for health promotion policy. The set of techniques which have been developed from the economic way of thinking are then described, followed by an illustration which shows the way that economic appraisal can help with decision making in health promotion.

ECONOMICS AS A WAY OF THINKING

Economics is the study of how society chooses to use its scarce resources to produce various outputs (goods and services). It is also about who benefits from those outputs. In economics, the term 'resources' refers to those things which contribute to production, such as land, labour, and equipment. Money only contributes to production if used to rent land, hire labour, buy equipment, etc. In other words money gives a command over resources, but is not itself a resource.

Within the formal health care sector, the production of 'better health' requires the input of various health service resources such as doctors, nurses, drugs, dressings, and operating theatres. In the case of much prevention, better health can also be viewed as something produced by individuals combining their own time with various other inputs.

The starting point of economics is that resources are scarce relative to the demands made on them. On a national level, it is not possible to double the output of all goods and services because of an insufficiency of available resources. Scarcity means that large increases in any one type of output may be achieved only by shifting resources away from the production of other outputs, thus sacrificing what would otherwise have been produced. In economic thinking the *cost* of any production is perceived in terms of these sacrifices, i.e. what has been forgone by not using the resources in another way. This is called 'opportunity cost' and is a different concept from money cost.

Opportunity cost is also a relevant concept when viewing the individual as a producer of his or her own health improvements. The time available to put into health production is finite, and the money available to command the other needed resources is also limited. A programme of exercise may not involve any monetary expenditure, but since the time spent exercising means forgoing benefits from work or leisure time, there is an opportunity cost.

Scarcity means that choices must be made about how to allocate resources between competing alternatives. While there can be no single basis on which all choices should be made, it is at least possible to identify a number of criteria for choice. The criterion most used in economics is 'efficiency', which is about attempting to maximize the benefits from available resources. According to this criterion it is unwise to devote resources to A if more benefit could be obtained by using the resources in B. If C and D produce the same level of benefit, but C does so using fewer resources, then C is the more efficient. One activity can never be said to be more efficient than another purely on the basis of being more beneficial or purely on the basis of being less costly. The decision must involve both.

Of course, maximizing benefits from available resources is not the only noble social objective. Inefficient policies can legitimately be pursued if other criteria, such as equity or political expedience, can justify them. Comparing programmes in terms of their efficiency, however, forces explicit identification and consideration of these other criteria if less efficient programmes are to be defended.

ECONOMICS AND HEALTH-AFFECTING BEHAVIOUR

As other chapters in this book demonstrate, theories have developed within various disciplines to explain health-affecting behaviour. Though economics is not conventionally thought of as a behavioural science, it contains a well-developed set of theories on what influences consumers' demand for various goods and services. If health-affecting behaviour is regarded as the demand for health-affecting goods and services, then economic theories of demand can provide an alternative explanation for such behaviour. Unfortunately, preventive goods (including preventive health care) and hazardous goods have attributes which complicate matters when they are analysed in terms of conventional demand theory.

In economic theory goods and services are demanded for the 'utility' (satisfaction) which they provide. Most health care services, however, do not directly yield positive utility. Health care can be unpleasant (can yield negative utility) and, unless we all have Munchausen syndrome, there must be some other explanation why people demand these services. Economists have postulated that the demand for health care is a 'derived demand'. People do not demand a health care service for its own sake. Rather, the demand for health care is derived from people's demand for health.

Clearly, the commodity 'health' is not something which only health care professionals can produce. In the preventive sense, individuals can produce health by combining their own time with various other resource inputs such as vitamin tablets, jogging shoes, or high-fibre cereals. (Note that in this context these goods are considered to be resources because they are contributing to production of something else.)

Based on the seminal work of Michael Grossman (1972), economists have developed models which see individuals as *producers* of health (see, for example, Cropper 1977; Ippolito 1981; Muurinen 1982). These are based on what is called the 'human capital' approach, in that individuals are seen as making new investments in their own health. These models have helped to increase our understanding of human behaviour regarding the demand for various preventive and hazardous goods. For example, while conventional demand theory explains and predicts how demand for a hazardous good such as cigarettes (or any other good) depends on its price, Ippolito's model shows how this demand is also dependent on whether the hazard is constant (i.e. has a fixed probability of death per unit consumed) or cumulative, as in the case of cigarettes.

Cohen (1984) has developed a model of preventive behaviour which differs from those above in its recognition that many preventive goods (and all hazardous goods) are not demanded for preventive reasons at all. According to this model, preventive or hazardous goods provide two types of utility – that derived directly from the use value of the good, e.g. the good taste of wholemeal bread or the pleasure of smoking, and that derived from the knowledge that consuming the good alters the risk of future illness or injury. This model provides messages for policy concerning the most effective way of manipulating the demand for preventive or hazardous goods. For example, the model suggests that advertising messages which address the use value of goods may be more effective than health education which focuses on risk attributes if the former are shown to dominate the decision to consume. In the case of smoking this may mean making smokers feel guilty about the annoyance they cause to non-smokers, rather than making them worry about their own future health.

As a means of explaining health-affecting behaviour, economics has not had a particularly great impact on the development of health promotion. This may in part be due to the presence of well-developed theories from other disciplines in this area. However, where economics is having a major influence on health promotion is in terms of evaluation.

ECONOMIC APPRAISAL

The cost-benefit approach, which is the foundation of economic appraisal, is outlined in Figure 6.1. The diagram shows that all policies/programmes/activities involve the use of resources. Whether these are resources diverted from other uses or made available for a specific use is irrelevant since in virtually all cases the resources could have been used in another way. The benefits of these other potential uses will be forgone if this programme is pursued. This sacrifice of benefits is the cost. At the same time something good must be expected to result. This is the benefit.

The cost-benefit approach is about weighing gains against sacrifices. Something passes the cost-benefit test if the value of the gains exceeds the value of the sacrifices. If it fails the test, the implication is that the required resources could produce greater benefit if used in another way. The trade-off is between benefits gained and benefits forgone, not between benefits gained and cash. Only in an ideal world of infinite resources could everything which produces benefit be pursued.

Costs can be defined as all resources which have alternative uses – hence which involve an opportunity cost. Benefits can be defined as all things of value which emerge. Non-resource costs such as anxiety or pain can be treated as negative benefits. Resource savings can be treated as negative costs. Not all exponents of the cost-benefit approach classify costs and benefits in quite this way (see, for example, Drummond 1980; Mooney et al. 1986). Nevertheless, there is no dispute about what factors need to be taken into account in an economic appraisal. How one separates costs and benefits

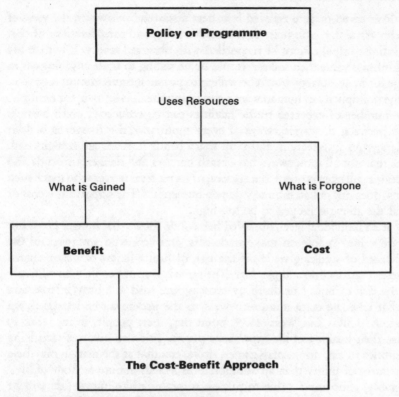

Figure 6.1   The cost-benefit approach
Source: Adapted from Drummond 1980

does not matter to the end result of the appraisal, so long as nothing of importance is omitted and the correct sign (+ or −) is applied.

The major problem of putting this theoretical framework into practice is of course that costs and benefits are not normally measured in common units. A list of costs and benefits will include such things as hours of doctor time, number of doses of a drug, and number of life years gained. As each of these is measured in different units, summing costs and benefits and then weighing one sum against the other is not possible unless a common unit can be found in which all can be described. Since, by definition, all costs and benefits have the common feature of being of value, and since the £ symbol represents relative value, it is possible (in theory at least) to express each in terms of its value and sum them accordingly.

Valuation is relatively straightforward when market prices are attached. If an ounce of gold sells for ten times more than an ounce of silver, it is normally accepted that gold is valued ten times more highly than silver. But how can a year of life be added to this comparison of values?

To many, the idea of even trying to put money symbols against benefits such as lives saved or pain relieved is at best distasteful. However, the view of those who argue that pain relief or human life is beyond considerations of cost (i.e. of infinite value) cannot be reconciled with observed reality. If human life were of infinite value then society would be unwilling to trade anything off in exchange for it, i.e. society would be willing to pay an infinite amount to save it. Given the multiplicity of human wants, this cannot be. It is known, for example, that the number of expected traffic fatalities can be reduced if crash barriers are built between the carriageways of every motorway, if a flyover is built at every dangerous intersection, and if all sharp bends in roads are straightened. The fact that not all motorways have crash barriers and dangerous bends and intersections still exist is proof that society, or its representatives who make such decisions, does not put an infinite value on human life. The opportunity cost of doing all the above is judged to be too high.

Even at an individual level, observed behaviour shows that human life is not of infinite value. People do make trade-offs. Smokers who are aware of the health hazard of smoking trade off the risk of future illness or death against their present satisfaction and pleasure. The same is true of people who willingly accept the risk of injury or death by crossing the road at a busy intersection rather that take the extra minute to walk to the pedestrian underpass down the road. As Cullis and West (1979) point out, 'Few people, if any, seek to maximise their health and life expectance per se. To do so involves sacrificing opportunities to eat, drink, play games, drive, etc. that at the margin may be a greater source of utility than an additional (expected) minute or hour of life.'

Inevitably, choosing a value to put on something like human life will be controversial, but such valuations cannot be avoided. Economists point out that they are made implicitly every time a decision either to do or not to do

Table 6.1 Some implied values of life

Source	Implied value of life
Screening of pregnant women to prevent stillbirth	£50
Government decision not to introduce childproof containers for drugs	£1,000
Motorway driving behaviour	£94,000
Legislation on tractor cabs	£100,000
Proposals for improved safety on trawlers	£1 million
Change in building regulations following collapse of Ronan Point high-rise flats	£20 million

Source: Adapted from Mooney (1977)

something is made. For example, if a motorway crash barrier programme is rejected on grounds of cost (say £X), and it is estimated that if it were constructed Y lives could be saved, then it is implied that the value of a life is less than £X/Y since this is what it would have cost on average to save each life.

Table 6.1 lists various implied values of life in different situations. In no case was this value made explicit at the time the decision was taken, yet the decisions implied values none the less. Since the people who may die in another Ronan Point disaster are unknown, i.e. they are statistical lives, and since the same is true for the babies not yet conceived whose lives could be save by screening of pregnant women, it must be asked why society is willing to spend £20 million to save a life in one area but unwilling to spend £50 to save a life in another. If the objective is to save the greatest number of lives (strictly it should be life-years) from the resources dedicated to life saving, then society's pursuit of this efficiency objective will be aided by this sort of information being available. There is nothing immoral about this.

Cost-benefit analysis

Cost-benefit analysis (CBA) begins by identifying and measuring in physical or other units all of the resources used or saved by the programme and all the positive or negative valued outcomes which result. It adopts what is called a 'social welfare' approach in which all costs and benefits are considered irrespective of who bears the costs or who receives the benefits. It then attempts to place money values on each. This allows CBA to answer the question of whether and to what extent any programme or policy should be pursued.

When market prices are available they are normally used to value costs and benefits. When market prices do not exist money values can still be applied by any of a variety of methods. The way in which money values can be placed on human life illustrates this.

The earliest method of valuing human life equated the value of a life with the productive potential of the individual. Narrow interpretation of this approach means that a value of zero must be placed on the lives of the elderly, the mentally handicapped, housewives, and others. The fact that health services (which have opportunity costs) are not withheld from these groups demonstrates that society clearly places a value greater than zero on their lives. Use of earning potential can, however, be defended by noting that *one* of the objectives of health care is to increase people's productivity. Valuations based on earning potential can then at least be viewed as minima. If someone who is kept alive and healthy will contribute £X to the economy, then society ought to be willing to pay at least £X to keep him or her alive to do it. This should not be interpreted as meaning that society should not be willing to spend £X+1.

A second method of assigning money values to human life is based on people's willingness to pay for small reductions in risk. While conceptually pleasing because it attempts to tease out the values of those actually at risk, the approach can be criticized on several grounds. For one thing the valuations which emerge are normally much higher than those estimated by other means (Jones-Lee 1976). For another, it is questionable whether individuals can attach any real meaning to a risk reduction from say 1 in 100,000 to 1 in 110,000 (Cohen 1981). Additionally, it is not clear whether consumer-based values are appropriate in health care valuation (Mooney 1986).

A third method is to use implied values as discussed above or to use the amounts which courts have awarded in compensation for accidental death. This method has merit in that it is based on existing decision-making procedures and value structures. The problem, as seen above, is that the range of values can be enormous.

Differential timing of costs and benefits

Shifting resources from one area to another, in particular from treatment to health promotion, can involve major changes in the timing of costs and benefits. Any shift from treatment to health promotion will involve forgoing current benefits for benefits which will arise in the future.

In financial appraisal, explicit recognition is given to the idea that society appears not to be indifferent to the timing of costs and benefits, preferring to delay costs as long as possible and receive benefits as soon as possible. This is expressed in the form of positive interest rates in financial markets. Discount rates (the inverse of interest rates) are applied to all future costs and benefits to express them in terms of their 'present values'. The treasury sets an official discount rate for all formal cost-benefit appraisals in the public sector. The rate is currently 6 per cent per annum in real (after adjusting for inflation) terms.

In theory, the same adjustment process is required for health costs and benefits. There is no dispute among economists on the validity of the discounting process. What is contentious is the choice of discount rate. Normally, the rate set by the Treasury is applied. In the case of health promotion, though, it can be argued that a lower rate should be applied, since the Treasury rate has the effect of reducing the present value of benefits which arise more than fifty years in the future to virtually zero. Since much health promotion is specifically undertaken with long time horizons in mind, such a severe adjustment can be argued to be inappropriate.

Non-economists may take a stronger line, arguing that the whole process of discounting is unjustified (West 1985). Failure to discount, however implies a 0 per cent discount rate which must be subject to the same demand for justification as any other. This would require defending the view that society is indifferent to sacrificing (say) ten lives today in exchange for the saving of ten lives in the future. Economists are unwilling to accept this argument, and all economic appraisals express costs and benefits in present value terms.

Dealing with uncertainty

Estimation of the benefits of health promotion programmes requires the use of assumptions – sometimes fairly heroic assumptions. Since the only thing certain about the future is that it is uncertain, this is inevitable. But what if these assumptions prove to be wrong?

Clearly, it is not possible for any technique to remove the problem of dealing with uncertainty. No technique can make the unknowable known, but, if it can indicate the extent to which getting each variable right matters, then much of value is gleaned.

Sensitivity analysis is a technique used within the cost-benefit framework to test how sensitive conclusions are to any changes in assumptions. It is applied by identifying those variables around which most uncertainty exists and altering their values. Essentially this means redoing the analysis using these altered figures. In many cases such changes make little difference to the overall result. In other cases changes can radically alter the original conclusion.

Sensitivity analysis gives an indication of the degree of confidence one can have in the conclusions. Additionally, it identifies which estimates and assumptions may require further investigation before a decision is taken.

Alternatives to cost-benefit analysis within the framework

Given the difficulties of assigning money values to intangibles, it is not surprising that full cost-benefit appraisals are rare. There are, however, a number of other techniques under the cost-benefit umbrella which are simpler to apply in practice. Inevitably, these are more restrictive in terms of how their conclusions can guide policy.

Cost-effectiveness analysis

By weighing gains against sacrifices CBA directly addresses the question of whether or to what extent any programme should be pursued. It questions the worth of the objective. Often, however, the question of whether to undertake or expand a programme is not at issue. A decision may already have been taken. The issue is no longer 'should we?', but *'how* should we?'. In such cases a simpler technique under the cost-benefit approach is available.

Cost-effectiveness analysis (CEA) accepts that there are normally alternative ways of pursuing any objective and seeks to find that alternative which either produces most benefit for a given cost or achieves a given benefit at least cost. Again a 'social welfare' view is adopted and the same definitions of costs and benefits apply. However, since an assessment of whether benefits *exceed* costs is not required, there is no need to place money values on benefits. Thus if a breast cancer screening programme is to be undertaken, CEA can indicate whether mammography is more *cost-effective* than thermography. CEA cannot say whether either form of screening is efficient.

The advantage of CEA is that benefits need only be expressed in 'units of effectiveness'. The disadvantage is that it can compare only alternatives which produce the given unit of effectiveness. This is not a problem with many programmes which have precise and clearly defined objectives. For examples, a breast cancer screening programme seeks to detect pre-symptomatic cancers. An appropriate unit of effectiveness could then be 'pre-symptomatic cancers detected'. A CEA would identify the method with the lowest cost per pre-symptomatic cancer detected. It would *not* seek the lowest cost per woman screened. 'Women screened' cannot be a unit of effectiveness because a screening method with a low cost per woman screened may fail to detect the cancers which are picked up by more expensive screening methods. It may be cheap, but not meet the objective at all.

In the case of much health promotion, however, there can be more than one objective (Engleman and Forbes 1986). For example, an anti-smoking promotion may have the objectives of 1) increasing knowledge and awareness to allow consumers to make more informed choices and 2) reducing smoking prevalence. A policy to increase tobacco duty may have the sole objective of reducing smoking prevalence (ignoring any incentives the government may have to raise more revenue). Which is more cost-effective?

If the chosen unit of effectiveness is 'number of people who quit' and the tax increase is shown to have the lower cost per quitter, then in this case the tax increase is the more cost-effective policy. But what about the benefits of a more informed population? Should this additional 'output' not also be taken into account? The answer is that it should, but CEA cannot do it. CEA does not allow for comparison of programmes with multiple outputs. This is not a problem with CBA.

This limitation to CEA should not imply that it has little place in the appraisal of health promotion. All that is required for increased use of CEA is an acceptance that the *principal* objective of health promotion is to achieve a healthier population. This allows health promotion to be compared with alternative means of achieving health gains – provided that the chosen units of effectiveness always are in terms of the output 'health'. In the examples above it would have to be accepted that stopping smoking and detecting pre-symptomatic breast cancers will reduce morbidity and mortality.

Any additional benefits which health promotion may confer can be dealt with in two ways. If a health promotion programme is shown to be a more cost-effective way of achieving a health gain, then any additional benefits need not be considered since their inclusion would only reinforce the conclusion already reached. They will only add icing to the cake. If health promotion is shown to be less cost-effective at achieving a health gain, then the implied value principle can now be employed. Anyone who still argues in favour of the health promotion programme must now explicitly value the additional benefits from the health promotion route at more than the difference in cost between the programmes.

For example, if increasing taxes has a cost per quitter of £100 and the health promotion programme has a cost per quitter of £120, then anyone arguing in favour of health promotion must be placing a value of at least £20 on the benefit of increased knowledge. What the 'correct' value for increased knowledge ought to be is not easily answered, but the appraisal has at least forced explicit consideration of this issue. If the tax route is chosen it will be implied that increased knowledge is worth less than £20. If the health promotion route is chosen it will be implied that it is worth at least £20. Note that this question of 'worth' is a cost-benefit not a cost-effectiveness issue. Further, economic appraisal does not answer the question. It mere provides the information to others who will make the decision.

Cost-utility analysis

The problem with cost-effectiveness analysis is that it can compare only programmes which produce the same units of effectiveness. It is thus arguably of value only within narrowly defined areas of activity. However, the broader is the chosen unit of effectiveness, the wider is the applicability of the results. For example, if one of the objectives of a programme is to save lives then choosing 'lives saved' (or more precisely years of life saved) as the appropriate unit of effectiveness will allow the cost per life saved in this programme to be compared with the cost per life save of any other life-saving programme.

While this broadening of cost-effectiveness analysis is useful, there remain two weaknesses. First, comparison is still limited to programmes whose benefits come in the form of life saving. Second, and perhaps more important, comparison by cost per life-year gained assumes that a year of life bedridden and in pain is equivalent to a year of life in perfect health. This problem could be overcome by using a 'global' measure which can describe the benefit from any health intervention. However, because the thing which it is measuring (health gain) is multidimensional and value laden, it will never be possible to derive a perfect global measure. It must be remembered, though, that the trade-off between health gains in one activity and health gains in another is unavoidable. If addressing the nature of these gains and losses by means of imperfect measures results in better decisions being taken, then the measures are of value. What is being sought is improvement not perfection.

In theory any intervention produces either of two basic benefit dimensions. It either makes people live longer or it improves the quality of their life, or some combination of the two. Thus in theory all interventions produce Quality Adjusted Life Years (QALY) (Rosser and Kind 1978). If the output of all programmes were measured in QALY terms, then comparison of cost/QALY would allow a complete generalization of cost-effectiveness analysis. This type of CEA using QALYs (or similar output measures) is called Cost-Utility Analysis (CUA).

A PRACTICAL EXAMPLE OF ECONOMIC APPRAISAL: GENERAL PRACTITIONER ADVICE TO QUIT SMOKING

Cigarette smoking is a major cause of preventable morbidity and mortality. It has been shown to be responsible for increased incidence of lung cancer, coronary heart disease, chronic bronchitis, emphysema, bladder cancer (Doll 1983), and Crohn's disease (Tobin *et al.* 1987). Smoking during pregnancy is associated with low birth-weight babies (Doll 1983) and childhood cancer (Stjernfeldt *et al.* 1986). Secondhand or passive smoking has been shown to increase risk of lung cancer in non-smokers (Wald *et al.* 1986) and of respiratory illness in children (Chen *et al.* 1986). Smoking is estimated to cost the NHS about £500 million per year and costs British industry about 16,000,000 lost working days valued at some £1,500 million in lost output (Cohen and Henderson 1988). The potential benefits from reduced cigarette smoking appear to be very large indeed.

The fact that potential benefits are large, however, is not sufficient reason to increase effort in this area. Evidence on a programme's ability to achieve these benefits is required, as is information on cost. Some preventable outcomes may not be major in terms of potential benefits, but if the benefits can be achieved at very small cost then programmes in this area may be more efficient than programmes directed at the larger morbidity and mortality areas.

The issue of reducing smoking prevalence can be addressed from either a cost-benefit or a cost-effectiveness approach. The former examines the extent to which anti-smoking measures are an efficient use of scarce resources: i.e. should more resources be directed to anti-smoking programmes? The second takes it as given that anti-smoking is a worthwhile pursuit and examines which alternative method of reducing smoking prevalence will achieve the greatest reduction at the least cost.

By the mid-1980s evidence was emerging to show that advice to smokers by their general practitioners on why and how they should quit could be an effective way of reducing smoking prevalence (Russell *et al.* 1979; Woods *et al.* 1980; Stewart and Rosser 1982; Wilson *et al.* 1982; Jamrozik *et al.* 1984; Richmond *et al.* 1986). Such advice, however, is not costless as it requires scarce general practitioner time, particularly if a repeat visit is part of the advice regime, as was the case in several of the cited studies.

Approach 1: cost-benefit analysis

A cost-benefit analysis of GP advice to stop smoking would identify all the resource costs of the programme. Based on current knowledge of the relationship between smoking and smoking related diseases, an estimate would be made of the expected reductions in these diseases. The benefits (and negative costs) of such reductions would be calculated under three broad headings: 1) resource savings from having to treat less smoking-related disease, and possibly from having to fight fewer fires – and the resulting losses of property and life; 2) productivity gains because the people not acquiring smoking-related diseases will not lose work and leisure time; and 3) all the intangible benefits of living a longer life and not suffering the pain and misery of illness. Expressing all costs and all benefits in money terms allows the cost-benefit test to be applied.

Smoking is a complex issue, however, and there are numerous problems in applying cost-benefit analysis in practice. Aside from the difficulty of assigning money values to the items under 3 above, a number of other questions arise. Should the 'utility loss' (the forgone pleasure) of ex-smokers be included? Should the annoyance caused to non-smokers by cigarette smoke be taken into account and what value should be place on it? Does smoking increase cleaning costs? If reduced smoking causes jobs to be lost in the tobacco industry do they have to be included?

Because of these and other complicating factors no one has yet produced a comprehensive cost-benefit study of anti-smoking programmes. It is not surprising, therefore, that GP advice in particular has not been put to the cost-benefit test.

Approach 2: cost-effectiveness analysis

General practitioner advice to stop smoking has the same objective as all other anti-smoking measures – to achieve a reduction in smoking prevalence which will bring about a reduction in smoking-related morbidity and mortality. There are other means of pursuing this objective, including:

— an increase in taxation
— a ban on smoking in public places/at work etc.
— a ban on advertising/sport sponsorship etc.
— stronger health warnings on cigarette packets
— restrictions on who can purchase cigarettes
— mass media anti-smoking campaigns.

There are arguments for and against each of these. Increased taxation is known to be effective. Estimates vary, but generally show that a 10 per cent increase in the real price of cigarettes (i.e after adjusting for inflation) will cause roughly a 4 per cent fall in cigarette consumption (Cohen and

Henderson 1988). One argument against increased taxation is that tobacco duty is a 'regressive tax' which hurts the poor more than the rich.

Bans on smoking in designated places can be considered an infringement on human rights (Tobacco Advisory Council 1981). Mass media health education may be less objectionable than bans because education is essentially only information which allows consumers to make informed choice. It has, however, been shown to be of rather limited effectiveness (Sumner 1971: Atkinson and Skegg 1973: Russell 1973; Peto 1974). Banning advertising of tobacco products is also of dubious effectiveness (Fujii 1980; Metra Consulting Group Ltd 1979; Johnson 1980) and outlawing tobacco sponsorship will arguably cause great harm to sport and the arts while having little effect on smoking prevalence.

Arguments for and against each of the methods above can be made from many perspectives including the sociological, psychological, ethical, and political. The economic perspective is not advocated as a superior way of thinking. It is only an alternative, but one which together with other perspectives can make a major contribution to health promotion.

Under the cost-effectiveness perspective the cost of each of the measures is estimated followed by estimates of the effectiveness of each in reducing smoking prevalence. A comparison is then made in terms of cost per quitter. The method with the lowest cost per quitter is the most cost-effective.

In the United States, Altman *et al.* (1987) compared the cost-effectiveness of three smoking cessation programmes aimed at smokers who had expressed a desire to quit: a self-help quit smoking kit; a smoking cessation contest with prizes; and a smoking cessation class. The quit rates achieved were 21 per cent for the kit, 22 per cent for the contest, and 35 per cent for the class. The marginal costs per quitter were $45, $61, and $266 respectively. Sensitivity analyses indicated that even if the effectiveness of the kit were to drop to a 6 per cent quit rate, it would still be the most cost-effective option. The clear implication was that, given a limited budget, a sufficient number of interested smokers, and an objective of maximizing the number of quitters, then spending the budget on the self-help kit would achieve the maximum smoking cessation.

Broadening the objective

While this is of help in choosing between anti-smoking programmes (and in the case above only between anti-smoking programmes aimed at smokers who have expressed a desire to quit), cost-effectiveness analysis is no more than a ranking of alternative ways of achieving a single objective; in this case getting people to quit smoking. In any ranking one of the alternatives must come out on top. The ranking tells us nothing about how efficient anti-smoking is *vis-à-vis* programmes which produce other types of benefits. It is of no help in choosing between anti-smoking and other activities.

One way of overcoming this is to extend the ranking by broadening the objective. Since reduced smoking will reduce mortality, the objective of GP advice to stop smoking can be couched in terms of life-years gained. If the alternative anti-smoking measures are compared in terms of cost per life-year gained, then the cost-effectiveness of each can be compared with the cost-effectiveness of any other programmes which produce benefits in the form of life-years gained.

A recent study by Cummings *et al.* (1989) measured the effectiveness of GP advice to stop smoking in terms of 'life years gained'. The cost per life-year from an original brief advice session ranged from $705 to $988 for men, and from $1204 to $2058 for women, depending on the assumptions used. The authors were able to compare this with the cost-effectiveness of other preventive measures which had been appraised in cost per life-year terms, including treating moderate hypertension ($11,300), treating mild hypertension ($24,408), and treating hypercholesterolemia ($65,000–108,000). Thus, a cost-effectiveness study using this broader unit of effectiveness allows comparisons beyond the specific area of non-smoking.

Further broadening the objective

While this broadening of cost-effectiveness analysis is useful, there remain the two weaknesses described earlier, viz. comparison is still limited to programmes whose benefits are in the form of life saving and there is an implied assumption that life-years of different quality are valued equally.

To overcome this, a cost-utility analysis of GP advice to stop smoking was undertaken by Williams (1990), which estimated the marginal cost per QALY (from reduced coronary heart disease alone) to be £167. One objective of this study was to exemplify the QALY approach, and despite his acknowledged need to make some fairly heroic assumptions, Williams was able to compare this figure with other programmes which have been appraised in terms of cost per QALY, such as pacemaker replacement for heart block (£700), kidney transplantation (cadaver) (£3000), heart transplantation (£5000), and hospital haemodialysis (£14,000).

It is important to stress that cost/QALY information is intended to assist, not replace decision making. It advises that resources shifted *on the margin* from high to low cost/QALY programmes will allow an overall increase in benefit at no additional resource cost, i.e. there will be an efficiency gain. Cost/QALY figures will vary as programmes are expanded or contracted and a high figure must not be interpreted as calling for an end to that programme. Williams' results imply that additional resources would be far more efficiently used to increase GP advice to smokers than to expand the hospital haemodialysis programme.

CONCLUSION

The main message from economics is that health promotion may well be a good thing but it should not be blindly pursued. The expected benefits of health promotion may be attractive, but no benefits are achieved without sacrifices.

As this book shows, health promotion comes in many forms and guises. As a discipline, economics contributes to health promotion by identifying which forms of health promotion are worthwhile and which are not. It provides a framework which enables identification of where the benefits of health promotion justify the cost and to what extent. Economics is about informed choice not evangelism.

This is an important aspect of health promotion because properly conducted economic appraisals present reasoned and justifiable arguments as to why more resources should be directed towards health promotion generally. In terms of dealing with competing health promotion programmes, economics can show how resources can be most cost-effectively allocated to ensure the maximum health gains from whatever level of resources is secured for these activities.

As a behavioural science, economics can also make an important contribution to health promotion by increasing our understanding of what affects health-promoting behaviour. There is much scope for increasing this contribution of economics in future.

REFERENCES

Altman, D. G., Flora, J. A., Fortmann, S. P., and Farquhar, J. W. (1987) 'The cost-effectiveness of three smoking cessation programs', *American Journal of Public Health* 77: 162–5.

Atkinson, A. B. and Skegg, J. L. (1973) 'Anti-smoking publicity and the demand for tobacco in the U.K', *Manchester School of Economics and Social Studies* 41: 265–82.

Chen, Y., Li, W., and Yu, S. (1986) 'Influence of passive smoking on admissions for respiratory illness in early childhoods', *British Medical Journal* 293: 303–6.

Cohen, D. R. (1981) *Prevention as an Economic Good*, Health Economics Research Unit, Discussion Paper No. 02/81, University of Aberdeen.

——(1984) 'The utility model of preventive behaviour', *International Journal of Social Economics* 10: 52–62.

Cohen, D. R. and Henderson, J. (1988) *Health, Prevention and Economics*, Oxford: Oxford Medical Publications.

Cropper, M. L. (1977) 'Health, investment in health, and occupational choice', *Journal of Political Economy* 86: 1273–94.

Cullis, J. G. and West, P. A. (1979) *The Economics of Health: An Introduction*, Oxford: Martin Robertson.

Cummings, S. R., Rubin, S. M., and Oster, G., (1989) 'The cost-effectiveness of counseling smokers to quit', *Journal of the American Medical Association* 261, 1: 75–9.

Doll, R. (1983) 'Prospects for prevention', *British Medical Journal* 280: 445–53.

Drummond, M. F. (1980) *Principles of Economic Appraisal in Health Care*, Oxford: Oxford Medical Publication.

Engleman, S. R. and Forbes, J. (1986) 'Economic aspects of health Education', *Social Science and Medicine* 22: 443–58.

Fujii, E. T. (1980) 'The demand for cigarettes: further empirical evidence and its implications for public policy', *Applied Economics* 12: 479–89.

Grossman, (1972) 'On the concept of health capital and the demand for health', *Journal of Political Economy* 80: 223–55.

Ippolito, P. M. (1981) 'Information and the life cycle consumption of hazardous goods', *Economic Inquiry* 19: 529–58.

Jamrozik, K., Vessey, M., Fowler, G., Wald, N., Parker, G., and Van Vanakis, H. (1984) 'Controlled trial of three different antismoking interventions in general practice', *British Medical Journal* 288: 1499–503.

Johnson, J. (1980) 'Advertising and the aggregate demand for cigarettes: a comment', *European Economic Review* 14: 117–25.

Jones-Lee, M. W. (1976) *The Value of Life: An Economic Analysis* London: Martin Robertson.

Metra Consulting Group Ltd (1979) *The Relationship Between Total Cigarette Advertising and Total Cigarette Consumption in the U.K.*, London: Metra Consulting Group.

Mooney, G. H. (1977) *The Valuation of Human Life*, London: Macmillan.

——(1986) *Economics, Medicine and Health Care*, Brighton: Wheatsheaf.

Mooney, G. H., Russell, E. M., and Weir, R. D. (1986) *Choices for Health Care*, 2nd edition, Basingstoke: Macmillan.

Muurinen, J. M. (1982) 'Demand for health: a generalised Grossman model', *Journal of Health Economics* 1: 5–28.

Peto, J. (1974) 'Price and consumption of cigarettes: a case for intervention?', *British Journal of Preventive and Social Medicine* 28: 241–5.

Richmond, R. L., Austin, A., and Webster, I. W. (1986) 'Three year evaluation of a programme by general practitioners to help patients to stop smoking', *British Medical Journal* 292: 803–6.

Rosser, R. and Kind, P. (1978) 'A scale of valuations of states of illness: is there a social consensus?', *International Journal of Epidemiology* 7(4): 347–58.

Russell, M. A. H. (1973) 'Changes in cigarette price and consumption in men in Britain, 1946–71: a preliminary analysis', *British Journal of Preventive and Social Medicine* 27: 1–7.

Russell, M. A. H., Wilson, C., Taylor, C., and Baker, C. D. (1979) 'Effects of general practitioner advice against smoking', *British Medical Journal* 2: 234–5.

Stewart, P. J. and Rosser, W. W. (1982) 'The impact of routine advice on smoking cessation from family physicians', *Canadian Medical Association Journal* 126: 1051–4.

Stjernfeldt, M., Berglund, K., Lindsten, J., and Ludvigsson, J. (1986) 'Maternal smoking during pregnancy and risk of childhood cancer', *Lancet* i: 1350–2.

Sumner, M. T. (1971) 'The demand for tobacco in the U.K.', *The Manchester School* 39: 23–36.

Tobacco Advisory Council (1981) *Advertising Controls and Their Effects on Total Cigarette Consumption*, London: TAC.

Tobin, M. V. *et al.* (1987) 'Cigarette smoking and inflammatory bowel disease', *Gastroenterology* 93: 316–21.

Wald, N. J., Nanchahal, K., Thompson, S. G., and Cuckle, H. S. (1986) 'Does breathing other people's tobacco smoke cause lung cancer?', *British Medical Journal* 293: 1217–22.

West, R. R. (1985) 'Valuation of life in long run health care programmes', *British Medical Journal* 291: 1139–41.

Williams, A. (1990) 'Screening for risk of CHD: is it a wise use of resources?', in M. Oliver, M. Ashley-Miller, and D. Wood (eds) *Strategy for Screening for Risk of Coronary Heart Disease*, London: Wiley.

Wilson, D., Wood, G., Johnston, N., and Sicurella, J. (1982) 'Randomized clinical trial of supportive follow-up for cigarette smokers in a family practice', *Canadian Medical Association Journal* 126: 127–9.

Woods, O. J., Cullen, M. J., and Dorman, R. H. (1980) 'The prevention of coronary heart disease in general practice', *Journal of the Royal College of General Practitioners* 30: 52–7.

Chapter 7

Health promotion as social policy

Robin Bunton

Health promotion professes to be centrally concerned with the social policy process. Building healthy public policy is one of the five means of health promotion action to achieve Health For All by the Year 2000 – along with creating supportive environments, strengthening community action, developing personal skills, and reorientating health services. To promote health effectively, we need to be able to understand, analyse, and ultimately influence social and health policy. Social policy should have a substantial input to health promotion, taking health promotion on its own terms. More than this, however, the study of social policy might contribute to our understanding of the emergence of health promotion itself. Health promotion has developed along with and in response to a social and political context particular to the late twentieth century. Understanding this social and political policy context, and health promotion's place in it, not only provides important self-awareness but allows a better understanding of the constraints on and possibilities for developing healthy public policy. Health promotion itself is a topic of interest to social policy analysts (Beattie 1991) and might be seen as an area of social policy. There are substantial areas of overlap between the two fields of study.

This chapter examines the contribution the study of social policy can make to the study of health promotion, and in particular to healthy public policy. It outlines the salient features of the academic study of social policy, its focus and perspective, and suggests how these might contribute to the study of healthy public policy. Substance misuse policy is examined illustratively, as an area of social policy that is also an area of healthy public policy concern. To do this it is first necessary to describe healthy public policy itself.

HEALTHY PUBLIC POLICY

Defining healthy public policy can be problematic due to both variation in use of the term and inherent conceptual ambiguity (Pederson *et al.* 1988). Though the term itself is a recent one, it can be seen to be a direct descendant of the public health movements prior to the 'new public health' and intimately linked to the development of World Health Organization programmes. The conceptual grounding for healthy public policy came from the WHO Assembly's resolution that health be the main social goal of government, including Health For All by the Year 2000. Subsequent conferences and concept statements have given substance to healthy public policy, as did the WHO conference on healthy public policy held in Adelaide (WHO 1988b) which produced the following definition:

Healthy Public Policy is characterized by an explicit concern for health and equity in all areas of policy and by an accountability for health impact.

The concept anticipates a new culture of public policy that is pluralistic and looks beyond state administrative planning structures to develop and implement policy, calling for multi-sectoral, multi-level, and participative initiatives.

A useful distinction has been made between healthy public policy and public health policy (Hancock 1982). The latter term refers to a narrower set of policies, more usually aimed at the system of caring for ill people. This distinction is a crucial one. Healthy public policy self-consciously aims to go beyond the health care system and its more traditional hospital and physician-based care. Definitions of healthy public policy incorporate very broad visions of health, crossing traditional disciplinary, organizational, and governmental categories. They refer to a concern for manipulating the social policy environment to create a healthy society, implicitly recognizing that the social environment is an important determinant of health. Milio's elegant definition captures this well, describing, healthy public policy as 'Ecological in perspective, multi-sectoral in scope and participatory in strategy' (Milio 1987). Being ecological and to some extent holistic, such an approach claims to recognize the complexity of the determinants of health and disease (Milio 1986). Various sectors of society are understood to act in interdependence to regulate, enhance, or endanger health. Governmental sectors outside health are involved in engendering health – agriculture, education, transportation, energy, and housing, for example.

Such an approach implies new ways of thinking about health and government policy and suggests the design of overarching mechanisms linking very different policy sectors. Governments should, it is argued, view health as a resource and plan to maximize its production by social and economic development. Central government mechanisms have been suggested that vet all policies for their health effect (or gain) in much the same way that policies are now vetted by treasury departments (Milio 1986). Mobilizing for the development of healthy public policy will require new organizational mechanisms and new means of co-ordination to bring about new alliances. New methods of working will also be necessary.

Though sometimes confused with health promotion policy, healthy public policy takes a broader focus than this neighbouring concept, which tends to refer to the development of specific health promotion programmes such as the development of no-smoking policies or healthy diet policies, or even the establishment of health promotion organizations or structures. Healthy public policy refers to multi-sectoral and collaborative processes involving the participation of all groups and populations affected.

Collaboration and co-ordination are needed to draw upon the wide range of activities needed to promote healthy public policy. Participation also features largely. If multi-sectoral collaborative efforts are to be achieved, then different sectors, groups, or communities must be made aware of the health consequences of their actions and be made to gain commitment to change. There has been a call for greater public accountability for health and the development of partnerships in the policy process. Slogans and catchphrases such as 'intersectoral planning', 'community participation', 'putting health on the agenda of policy makers' abound and have become synonymous with the Health For All by the Year 2000 movement. Corporate and business interests, non-government bodies, and community organizations all have potential for preserving and promoting people's health. This aspect of mobilizing for healthy public policy is perhaps the most challenging and will involve enabling and empowering of larger sections of the community (Stacey 1988). It is also an area most lacking in theory and research (Pederson et al. 1988) and may be an area in which social policy analysis has much to offer. Understanding how groups and organizations come to act upon and change aspects of their everyday world is central to understanding the healthy public process.

The Adelaide Conference on healthy public policy identified a number of areas for immediate action. It recognized that equity and access to health resources – health care, healthy environments, and other health-enhancing goods and services – are fundamental to promoting and protecting health. Four areas were prioritized: the health of women, food and nutrition, tobacco and alcohol, and the creation of supportive environments. New alliances are recommended as a means of achieving such action, such as the joining of public health and ecological movements locally, nationally, and internationally. Commitment to global health is central to these re-commendations. There is an inherent refusal to take as given the social policy environment, along with a call for changes in the social and political environments.

The development of the concept of healthy public policy stresses the need to understand and analyse the policy environment in a very broad sense. It points to the need for analysis of broader beliefs and cultures as well as detailed understanding of the nature of available policy advocates, areas of public support, the nature of key 'stakeholders' and influencers of policy, as well as government and organizational structures. Such an area of study could be said to form the *raison d'être* of social policy. The broad focus of concern matches that of the contemporary discipline, though this has not always been the case. There would appear to be a substantial convergence of interest between health promoters and social policy analysts at least as far as the area of study is concerned. Perspectives may vary considerably within health promotion, as this book illustrates. Variety also exists in the study of social policy, as the following brief outline of the discipline illustrates.

SOCIAL POLICY

Social policy refers to the sets of arrangements and structures associated with state policies, ranging from broad economic policy to specific areas such as crime control. Social policy is more often used to refer to policies which are 'integrative' in one way or another; that is, they are designed to bind or bring about harmonizing society in one way or another (Boulding 1967).

Though usually associated with national and local government, social policy may be the result of non-government initiatives or the unintented outcome of a variety of political, social, and organizational imperatives. Social policy also refers to a particular field of academic study, with its own concerns and perspectives. It is the academic study of social policy that is the main concern of this chapter, though these two areas cannot easily be divorced from one another. The study of social policy is in large part influenced by current developments in the social policy environment. In discussing the academic discipline of social policy, therefore, it will be necessary and useful to refer to recent changes in the social policy environment.

Seen as a discipline, in the loose sense of the term used throughout this volume, social policy is a relatively new one. It emerged very much (along with its allied discipline social administration) in response to unprecedented expansion of the welfare state in the late nineteenth and early twentieth centuries, providing an academic background for the emerging social service occupations (Brown 1983). The subject grew with a distinct institutional focus, studying the nature of a rapidly growing social service provision. In Britain, like many other Western or Northern societies, the end of the Second World War marked a new era of welfare administered either by central or local government, which replaced the piecemeal provision of the nineteenth and early twentieth centuries. General social services became an integral part of state activity attempting to eliminate the so-called 'five great areas of want': poverty, homelessness, ignorance, disease, and idleness (unemployment). In Britain, a number of blue-print type documents such as the Beveridge report (Beveridge 1942) appeared, shaping the construction of the welfare state. The introduction of national insurance schemes, family allowances, national assistance, national health services, state education, and children's welfare systems were commonly developed along with local government housing.

The study of social policy reflected these concerns. Marshall, one of the founders of the discipline, defined social policies by their welfare objectives – security, health, and welfare. He contrasts such policies with economic policies which are less altruistic. Social policies, he has argued, are concerned with collective interventions to promote individual welfares, often using political power to supersede or modify the operations of the economic system (Marshall 1975). Marshall distinguished three aims of social policies: the elimination of poverty, the pursuit of equity, and the maximization of welfare. The study of social policy was intimately linked to reforms on all these fronts and has been dubbed 'the book-keeping of reform' (Rex 1978). Key individuals within the discipline in Britain have been linked to Fabianism and explicitly committed to social reform (Brown 1983).

The focus of social policy is much broader than these concerns, however, and also more critical. Titmuss, another important founder and the first Professor of Social Administration, defined his subject as the study of eight areas:

1 The analysis and description of policy formation and its consequences, intended and unintended.
2 The study of structure, function, organization, planning and administrative processes of institutions and agencies, historical and comparative.
3 The study of social needs and of problems of access to, utilization, and patterns of outcome of services, transactions, and transfers.
4 The analysis of the nature, attributes and distribution of social costs and diswelfares.
5 The analysis of distributive and allocative patterns in command-over-resources-through-time, and the particular impact of the social services.
6 The study of the roles and functions of selected representatives, professional workers, administrators and interest groups in the operation of social welfare institutions.
7 The study of the social rights of the citizen as contributor, participant and user of the social services.
8 The study of the role of government (local and central) as an allocator of values and of rights to social property as expressed through social and administrative law and other rule-making channels.

(Titmuss 1968 quoted in Brown 1983)

This description, demanding though it is, does not exhaust the concerns of the subject. Social policy is not simply concerned with the analysis and critique of administrative institutions and processes and the effects of government welfare policies. It is also interested in the structures and processes of wider society which create a given distribution of resources, have a bearing on welfare, and, in turn, regulate the institutions which manage that distribution (Walker 1983). All areas of government policy can influence social policy, including 'the social purposes and consequences of agriculture, economic, manpower, fiscal, physical development and social welfare policies' (Rein 1970). Broader societal structures of kinship, social groups, occupational structures, fiscal structures, and many other organizing principles of society have an influence over welfare and social policy. It is, for example, difficult to conceive of the Western state as existing entirely separately from industry and financial institutions. In most capitalist societies the two are intimately linked. Rather than see social policy as attempting to modify the play of market forces, as Marshall suggested, social policy might be seen to be organized to suit the vested financial interests represented through the political system. The industrial sector has an important influence over social inequalities. The state can respond to this in a number of ways. Low pay, for example, has consistently been responsible for significant levels of poverty. Policies to counter this may be aimed to improve the incomes of those workers by tax incentives or income supplements; governments may also develop minimum wage policies. The state can also attempt to influence the industrial structure itself. Governments are important purchasers of goods and service and can influence industrial development by regulation of the location of industry and by other means.

Social structure may act to limit or undermine social policies to promote equity. Policies to reduce poverty, for example, may run up against fundamental class differences that not only restrict attempts to introduce a more equitable distribution of resources, but also influence and restrict policies designed to do so. Welfare policies cannot be discussed in isolation from a critique of the social structure (Walker 1983) nor from accounts of the social construction of social policy. There is a need to look at the forces and power relations that underpin the formation of social policies. Such an approach focuses on the functions and outcomes of social policy typical of a number of analysts (Titmuss 1974; Townsend 1975). Social policy examines, then, the rationale and underlying ordering principles which affect the distribution of resources, status, and power between different groups and individuals in society.

Examples of social policy, and its place in broad social structures, can be seen in analysis of health policy. The place of medical welfare, it has been suggested, promotes particular class interests within capitalist societies (Navarro 1976). Other powerful interests have been dominant in the development of medical and other welfare provision, such as the influence of professional groups (Freidson 1970; Wilding 1982). Recent developments in health policy may be restricting and challenging such interests (Elston 1991). Critiques of such power have influenced the development of health promotion and the new public health (Ashton and Seymour 1988). It has also led to recommendations to develop policies on the professions.

The place of the state as one of the main policy-forming bodies has received much discussion within social policy. As a potential regulator of social structure, the state has opportunity to control and regulate as well as to provide security and protection. The fate of particular groups can be influenced in both directions. Feminists, for example, have been ambivalent because of such propensities. On the one hand, the state can assist women to develop new forms of interdependence based in the community and not in more 'repressive' family structures. Community child care initiatives, hostels, employment, and education for women may act in this way, for example, and can strengthen women's interests and counter patriarchal interests. At the same time, however, state provision may have its own repressive functions and serve the needs of capitalism in other ways; it can construct its own version of family life and values which do not suit the needs of women (Fitzgerald 1983; Wilson 1983). State policy has the potential to regulate particular social groups or even to marginalize them (Small 1988; Pascall 1986; Manning 1985). Such dangers exist in areas of healthy public policy also. Introducing new forms of communication, co-ordination, inter-sectoral and inter-agency liaison in effect introduces new social regulation technologies. There are dangers in manipulation of such mechanisms, resulting in new forms of social control (Bunton 1990; Evers *et al.* 1990).

Social policy then has a very broad range of interests, examining the values, principles, and rationales that govern distribution of resources and the formation of policies on the one hand, whilst being interested in the impact of such principles on social relationships, behaviours, organizations, professions, classes, on the other. Such a broad remit requires a broad intellectual base and social policy has developed drawing on a range of disciplines.

The eclectic base has also been matched with a empiricist tradition. A strong research programme directed at the analysis of social need, social problems has been a feature of the subject from its inception. A concern for research methodology, field work, and survey analysis has been dominant. Topics such as poverty and ill health, child neglect and housing have remained common concerns.

POLICY PROCESS

Social policy is centrally concerned with the processes of policy formation. Questions about how policy development can be brought about more efficiently have concerned the discipline, as they do health promotion. Policy studies is an allied field of study that is drawn upon in this area. Policy itself has been well defined by Blum:

> Policy is a long-term, continuously used standing decision by which more specific proposals are judged for acceptability. It is characterized by behavioural consistency and repetitiveness on the part of those who make it and those who abide by it.
>
> (Blum 1981)

This definition refers to decisions made over time. Similarly, policy has been conceived as a web of decisions (Easton 1953) and a process of decisions (Widavsky 1979). We might also conceive of different competing and interacting policies or systems of policy making.

Analysis of content seeks to describe and explain the genesis and development of particular policies. Much of UK academic study of social policy has
been conducted in this way. The process of identification of social problems
which social policies address is an identifiable area of study in itself (Manning
1985). Changes in policy over time can be plotted in a number of areas.

The nature of the 'social liquor' problem, for example, has changed
significantly over time (Makela and Viikari 1977). Late nineteenth- and
early twentieth-century concerns, motivated, amongst other things, by
attempts to instil bourgeois self-discipline in the newly industrialized
working class (Harrison 1971; Gusfield 1963; Blocker 1976), culminated in
early twentieth-century temperance movements which aimed to restrict and
control the product, alcohol. Following the political failure of prohibition,
emphasis shifted to the individual aspects of the problems associated with
addiction. A concern for 'alcoholism' characterized policy from the 1930s to
the mid-twentieth century. By the late twentieth century, a 'post addiction'
approach had emerged, drawing upon behaviourally and environmentally
conceived problems and fitting within a public health perspective on alcohol
problems (Room 1981; Berridge 1989). Policy on illicit drugs has gone
through similar changes (Stimson 1987), though shifting significantly in the
1980s and 1990s in response to policy on HIV/AIDS (Berridge 1990). Such
change can be found in many areas of healthy public policy.

Policy analysis also focuses on the stages through which policy action
passes, attempting to account for the influences on these processes which
may be societal, governmental, organizational, or even individual. Any
analysis of the policy process can be broken down into component parts.
A sevenfold typology is preferred by several authors (Hogwood and Gunn
1981; Gordon et al. 1977; Ham and Hill 1984), referring to: policy content,
policy process, outputs, evaluation studies, information for policy making,
process of advocacy, and policy advocacy.

Policy content seeks to describe and explain the genesis and development
of particular policies. Much of UK social policy has been conducted in this
way. Policy process focuses on the stages through which policy action passes
and attempts to assess influences upon this process(es). Such analysis may
be directed at organizational, governmental, or societal processes. A third
area of study is that of policy outputs which seeks to explain the variety
of levels of expenditure or service provision. Policies may be examined
as dependent variables influenced by social, economic, technological, and
other variables (Dye 1976). Evaluation or impact studies are concerned
with the impact policies have on a population. Fifthly, there is information
for policy making which is the method of amassing information to assist
policy makers in reaching decisions. This may be carried out by government
departments, academics, or other organizations. Process advocacy refers to
attempts to improve the nature of the policy-making system, particularly the
machinery of government through the development of planning systems and

new approaches to co-ordination which involve the analyst in pressing for
specific options and ideas in the policy process, either on their own behalf
or via a pressure group. Within this sevenfold typology, a distinction can be
made between policy analysis which provides a more academic or objective
understanding *of* policy (the first three) and one which provides more
committed analysis *for* policy development (the latter three). On the whole
the literature on healthy public policy falls into the category of committed
policy analysis.

Understanding of the implementation process is central to understanding
any policy development. The adoption of particular policies by different
groups and subcultures will depend on how such policies are conceived,
how they are introduced, the group's commitment to them, the local
resources available to assist their introduction, and a range of other
socio-economic factors. Policies and strategies can be modified and altered,
often substantially, during development. The presence of powerful interests
can have an obstructive or 'watering down' effect in such cases (Hawks
1990). It has become apparent that policy introduction conceived of only
as a 'top-down' process is very limited in health promotion (Donati 1988).
Policy development can also be generated from the 'bottom-up' and success
might depend upon a combination of top-down and bottom-up approaches
(Sabatier 1986). Context will affect all implementation, and understanding
of macro and local power structures within the socio-political environment
is central to success (Barrett and Hill 1984; Milio 1987).

Central to the implementation of healthy public policy is the development
of co-ordinating mechanisms to facilitate multi-sectoral involvement and
community participation. Co-ordination might be achieved by the establishment of a central body or organization or, alternatively, by enabling
local bodies working on single issues. In any co-ordination, there will
be key decision makers and resource allocators to be identified and key
'stakeholders' who will influence the course of policy co ordination. Analysis
of the policy process must take account of these factors in building a picture
of the policy context.

A large number of factors come to bear on the policy process. Analysis of
these policy contexts will be central to assessing the feasibility of developing
healthy public policy. This analysis will clarify the limitations and constraints
placed on any policy development. Much will depend on this analysis. If the
study of social policy has much to offer here, it offers this in competing forms
of analysis. Interpretation of macro and micro social, political, and economic
structural process is complex and there are a variety of perspectives on the
best way to do so.

PERSPECTIVES

Theoretical differences and diverse models or perspectives have always been a part of social policy. Difference and diversity have become much more accented in the latter decades of the twentieth century, which have been characterized by much theoretical ferment and change – much of this in response to a rapidly changing political focus in the policy environment.

Debates had taken place in academic circles in the late 1960s over the appropriateness of state interventions. Some favoured 'universal' provision of social welfare as a basic right of citizenship (Townsend 1968; Titmus 1968; Redding 1970), whilst others argued for more limited 'selective' interventions for the needy only (Friedman 1962; Gray and Sheldon 1969). By the early 1970s there were signs of a breakdown in consensus within social policy which was to reflect broader ideological debate. Questions had been raised about the whole principle of social care mechanisms, asking: how far had they succeeded? who benefited from them? whose interests had social policies serviced? and what influenced their operation? This discussion coincided with broader socio-political change and what has been referred to as a 'crisis' in welfare. Economic changes and problems of the mid-1970s – inflation, recession, and low growth – had affected many Western societies and forced a rethink of welfare provision and in some cases an attack on the welfare state. There had been a tacit retreat from a commitment to welfare in Britain as early as the 1960s. Labour party policy had withdrawn from Keynesian approaches to economic regulation as the USA, Canada, and much of Europe was also to do in the face of a world economic recession (Loney et al. 1988). Public spending received substantial cuts.

Neo-conservative policies dominated the political agenda in Britain and the USA, providing ideological support for removing state spending and introducing measures to reduce what was seen as unnecessary state encroachment into the market and the lives of individuals. Income taxation was reduced, markets de-regularized, and state monopolies removed. A period of 'neo-liberal' government had begun which saw a changed role for the state, characterized by a rolling back of the state and a promotion of entrepreneurship and the market. There was a renewed belief in the market as a rational organizing principle which could successfully produce services sensitive to the needs of the consumer and successfully generate employment. Emphasis was placed upon self-reliance and initiative and avoidance of what was seen as the 'dangers' of dependency upon state provision. Neo-liberal concerns have been reflected in more recent social policy. The transformation in the social and economic underpinnings of welfare posed new problems and unearthed new study areas for the discipline. New sources of theory were drawn upon from sociology and political science in particular.

The mid-1970s saw new theoretical developments in British social policy in particular which led to more pronounced differences in perspective. George and Wilding (1976) were amongst the first to describe different ideologies of welfare in social policy. Though before this individual authors had been identified as having different 'values', these positions had not been patterned nor had their relevance been brought to the forefront of study. Analysis of ideology at once introduced the notion of social policies being the outcome of conflict and interests, and authors such as George and Wilding were critical of previous, often unacknowledged, consensus models of society where it was often assumed that policy developed rationally towards largely agreed upon objectives. This approach to public policy may be described as a 'rational deductive' and/or an 'incrementalist' approach (Ziglio 1987). By contrast, Marxist political economy, conflict, and pluralistic approaches were being put forward to provide understanding of the policy process.

There are a number of ways of representing the different ideological groupings of social policy analysts. George and Wilding's book is a good source of these, though there are others (Lee and Raban 1983). Understanding of these is an essential component of understanding social policy. One of the most common themes in such descriptions is pro- and anti-state positions. Analysts can be placed along a continuum according to these positions. George has identified a number of analysts constructing such types (George 1981).

Their various positions range from out-and-out free market individualists at one extreme to out-and-out collectivists in favour of the command economy at the other. More or less liberal and socialist collectivists in favour of the welfare state are arranged in the middle of the continuum. Each ideological grouping has, and spells out, a different set of expectations of and obligations upon states and upon citizens in the working of welfare provision and policy. Each set of prescriptions can be found in various forms in contemporary policy discussions.

Though applicable as a general sketch, we must be aware that there may be more subtle differences even within the various positions on this continuum. A useful distinction has been made between types of state intervention, between the state as a financer of welfare provision, a deliverer of welfare, and a regulator of welfare (Le Grand 1982). These analytic distinctions make ideological categorization a potentially complex exercise. All approaches to policy however will adopt a particular theoretical perspective (or set of perspectives) either explicitly or implicitly. A lack of awareness of the diversity in perspective may itself be a barrier to policy planning and implementation (Pederson et al 1988). Different groups may promote different policies at different times and for different reasons. Understanding this diversity is part of understanding the policy environment. Such diversity is readily identifiable in many healthy public policy initiatives. The rest of this chapter will examine some differences in positions within substance misuse policy which are illustrative of this. Within analysis of substance misuse

Figure 7.1 Typologies of welfare ideologies

PRO-
STATE

ANTI-
STATE

	Anti-Collectivism	Reluctant Collectivism	Fabian Socialism	Marxism[1]	
	Market Liberals	Political Liberals	Social Democrats	neo-[2] Marxists	
	Classical Economic Theory	neo-Mercantilism	Marxisms[3] 'its socialist derivatives'		
	Residual	Institutional	'Normative' or 'Socialist'[4]		
	Conservatism	Positive State	Social Security State	Social Welfare State	Radicalism[5]

Notes
1 George and Wilding (1976).
2 Room (1979).
3 Pinker (1979).
4 Mishra (1977: 35-6) and George and Manning (1980), after Titmuss (1974: Ch. 2).
5 Furniss and Tilson (1977).

Source: Lee and Raban 1983

policy, for example, there are those who work with a model that emphasizes conflict and confrontation of interests, whilst others would seem to adopt a more consensual view of policy planning and implementation. These will be examined respectively.

VARIETIES OF HEALTHY PUBLIC POLICY

Conflict

Most contemporary perspectives on drug misuse are associated with the 'new public health' and place emphasis on primary care, prevention, and health promotion. Problems are seen to be the result of various mixes of host, agent, and environment or, alternatively expressed, people, products, and settings (Robinson 1989). A problematic interrelation of three elements results in drinking and driving for example. Solutions to problems take place on a broad front and calls are made for an increasingly ambitious range of interventions (Chapman-Walsh 1990; Bunton 1990), some methods having a more proven track record than others (Grant 1989). Most of the current efforts have been geared to reducing consumption by depressing demand, though efforts have also been directed at supply (WHO 1988a). Though there are many potential fronts for health promotion related to drug misuse, those working within the field tend to prefer and emphasize one approach, rather than the whole range of possible interventions, revealing particular theoretical orientations.

A conflict or political economy approach to policy is more likely to favour state interventionist solutions to the problems relating to substance misuse. Such a conflict model would see fundamental oppositions of interests as a necessary part of the social order. Conflict theory has flourished in sociology (referred to in Thorogood's chapter) and has contributed much to the analysis of social policy. It has contributed much to the sociology of health and illness (Navarro 1976, 1982, 1986; Waitzkin 1983; Gerhardt 1989) and highlights oppositions of interests between producers and suppliers on the one hand and consumers on the other. This obvious division of interest is most starkly highlighted in relation to policy development on illegal drugs. Most societies have formulated policy on substance use that rests on assumptions of a fundamental opposition of interest between producers and consumers. Typically, this involves identifying some psychoactive substances that may legitimately be used and others that may not, without being subjected to sanction or punishment. There is great variety in the drugs brought under policy regulation in this way, even within Western societies. There are levels of agreement internationally however, witnessed by international efforts to suppress the use of heroine since the turn of the twentieth century (Hartnoll 1989). Subsequent efforts have been made to introduce control mechanisms.

Efforts are made nationally and internationally to prevent production and distribution (or 'trafficking'). Steps have been taken to seize financial assets of producers and distributors (or 'dealers'). A number of international bodies involved in the control of certain types of drugs have emerged, including the Commission on Narcotic Drugs (CND), the Division of Narcotic Drugs (DND), The International Narcotics Board (INCB), the United National Fund for Drug Abuse Control (UNFDAC), and Departments of the World Health Organization. Interpol and other international law enforcement mechanisms have also appeared.

Individual countries have developed policies, research studies, and enforcement mechanisms based upon a need to protect consumers or potential consumers from the dangers of exposure to specific sets of substances. Australia and the United Kingdom have both developed comprehensive drug strategies which have exhibited this exclusionary or restrictive policy. Opiates have been singled out for such restriction from most countries, though other substances, such as cannabis, have more frequently received a more lenient or liberal form of regulation (MacGregor 1989). There is some indication that efforts to reduce HIV/AIDS infection have had a liberalizing effect on policy towards injectable drugs in the UK (Berridge 1989: MacGregor 1989).

Public health policy on substance misuse have generally incorporated control and exclusion statements. The statement endorsed by the Adelaide Conference on healthy public policy is one such example of this (WHO 1988a). Whilst calling for measures to reduce demand, such as restriction of advertising and price increases, it also recommends regulating or eliminating the production of psychoactive substances and restricting availability of alcohol, tobacco, and other drugs through methods such as liquor licensing, street-level law enforcement, and rational prescribing practices.

Tobacco production is an area in which opposing interests and conflict in the policy process have been identified, representing a mismatch of interest between consumer and producer. World manufacture of tobacco products is controlled by a handful of multinational companies – the transnational tobacco conglomerates (TCCs) such as British American Tobacco and Imperial. These few companies effectively control most aspects of the business process – from leaf production to marketing and distribution of the final products (Booth *et al* 1990). TTCs have interests in paper mills, shipping, oil companies, retail networks, and are able to use all of these networks to ward off competition, to enter and develop new markets, and to influence price and quality. With such large corporate interests at stake the potential for creating health promoting environments may seem highly problematic. The power of tobacco producers and their ability to thwart efforts of advocates of public health policy has been well documented (Taylor 1984). Such analysis has often called for state intervention to curtail the play of market forces (whether these are seen as 'free enterprise' or monopolistic). The need to counterbalance the powers of the producer in the name of public health has also been well documented in relation to alcohol misuse.

Whilst many contemporary analysts of public policy on alcohol have tried to distance themselves from the highly centralized control of the temperance period, concern for aspects of production and distribution of alcohol has remained important to public health advocates (WHO 1988a). Debate about the role of the state in the regulation of production has pointed to fundamental conflicts of interest (Koskikallio 1979; Makela and Viikari 1977; Parker 1977). States must balance economic interests on the one hand against public health concerns on the other. This is not simply the opposition between commercial and public interest; the state itself is often a beneficiary of tax revenue from sales on alcohol. There may be internal conflict between different government departments. Despite state intervention, measures have been recommended on a wide number of fronts, including increasing relative price, restricting distribution to certain times, places, or social groups (e.g. age limits), increasing probability of detection and punishments for alcohol-related crime infringements (e.g. drinking and driving or public drunkenness), and numerous other policy measures (Grant 1989: Royal College of Physicians 1987: Home Office 1987a). Some countries have attempted to solve such conflicts by placing production and distribution of alcohol in the hands of the state monopolies, notably Sweden and Norway (Davies and Walsh 1983).

Substance misuse, then, would seem to highlight one area of healthy public policy where intransigent interests are a major obstacle to policy development. Consumer movements and co-operatives with aims closer to those of public health advocates frequently encounter the full force of such interests (Senoda 1990). Other areas of conflict of interests have been identified, however. It may be that fundamental inequalities in resources and power in society will continue to undermine attempts to work to agreed healthy public policy targets. Rhetoric on healthy public policy may have underestimated underlying conflict in this respect (Pederson et al. 1988) and could be accused of the idealism found in other Health For All statements (Strong 1986). Whilst such statements offer a positive starting point to policy development, there is a danger of glossing over differences in perspective that will imply differences in policy content, process, evaluation, and advocacy.

Some areas of healthy public policy may be appropriately placed within a combative or 'war oriented' model of making (Van der Kamp 1990). Structural conflict may be so fundamental to a social system that capital will almost always confront state and/or public interests. Inequalities in resources between state, capital, and civil society (including consumers and producers) may be such that policy options for health are severely limited. The social policy environment may be such that resource allocation prevents groups becoming involved in the policy-making process. Recent

UK trends towards greater differences between the rich and the poor is likely to exclude many people and groups from participation, or at least bias any input to the policy process (Farrent and Taft 1990). In other words, structural inequalities may shape and influence the policy process. In such circumstances, healthy public policy development may be less about challenging such inequalities than about developing better coping strategies and mechanisms, such as stronger community lobbies (Legg and Sylvan 1990). Analysis of these structures will largely determine the nature of one's perspective.

As well as being caused by structural inequality and imbalances of power, conflict can be generated by oppositions between forces of change and resistance to social innovation. Much health promotion effort is geared to developing techniques to enhance 'persuasive strategies' and to involve potential co-operators in policy change. In all the above senses, conflict may prove to be an important part of health promotion.

Consensus

The combative approach to healthy public policy is certainly not universal. For theoretical and empirical reasons, a number of analysts have emphasized the role of co-operation and collaboration. Much of the work on healthy public policy has demonstrated the potential for pooling of efforts (Evers *et al*. 1990). It has been argued that a different style and culture of public policy are emerging in health and social care which are pluralistic in approach and involve a greater number of actors than previously. 'Public' increasingly means more than state, and administrative planning is increasingly emerging from outside professional, government, or commercial quarters. The field of policy on substance misuse provides useful examples here also, often stressing the potential for efforts at the margins of economic and political institutions. Research in the field of alcohol policy, and UK policy on alcohol misuse in particular, can illustrate such an approach.

Two recent actions characterize the government's position. One of these was the establishment of an interdepartmental Ministerial Committee on Alcohol Misuse, established to review and co-ordinate government strategy (Home Office 1987b). The second was a clear declaration of government policy in the form of a circular calling for locally co-ordinated, multi-sectoral action to assess the extent of alcohol misuse and design methods of combating it, drawing upon local resources (DHSS 1989). The circular matches healthy public policy's exhortations to multi-sectoral multi-actor efforts. A feature of the government response has been the encouragement of involvement by the drinks trade to take steps to combat alcohol misuse, attempting to step up voluntary agreements on regulation and to introduce innovative schemes. This policy position reinforced earlier statements that talked of alcohol misuse being 'everybody's business' and called for:

> preventative action in which Government, the health professions and institutions, the business sector and trade unions, voluntary bodies and the people of the United Kingdom as individuals can all recognize and play their separate part.
>
> (DHSS 1981: 40)

The Government's position has been criticized for failing to grasp the nettle and introduce centralized fiscal measures to control consumption. It is accused of opting for what were seen as ameliorative steps, of seeing 'health education as the key to the problem' (Kendell 1987).

Over a similar period there were moves to relax central control mechanisms, such as the regulation of drinking hours (Home Office 1987b). These moves might well be seen to fit a new policy environment in which societal welfare solutions are being sought outside state intervention (Van Lennep 1980; Makela *et al.* 1981).

The case has been made for developing policy without putting exclusive efforts into the development of a national, or even global, co-ordinated policy initiative. Though some countries have been able to work towards such a plan (Australia, for example), concentration at this level can divert attention from the wealth of 'prevention potential' lying outside traditional state-centred control mechanisms. Rather than push for overall national objectives, efforts might be more productively aimed at 'what's already there' as policy resources (Maynard and Robinson 1990; Robinson 1989). Such an approach assumes certain levels of consensus can be achieved by drawing together different organizations and agencies with different interests and agendas through a process of 'partisan mutual adjustment' (Lindblorn 1965; Harrison and Tether 1990). Agreements may be reached through negotiation, bargaining, and manipulation. Diverse inter-organizational interests can be picked and matched to approxmiate something like overall policy.

The task of social policy in such research work is to explore areas of potential 'mutual adjustment' in order to maximize prevention potential in the cause of healthy public policy. This may well mean an extensive exploration of the complexity of the complete policy networks – from exploration of government departments and sub-departments and their responsibilities and decision-making powers (Harrison and Tether 1990) to the structure of the brewing trade (Booth *et al.* 1990; Grant 1989). The relative effectiveness of different regulatory mechanisms would need to be assessed within the policy complex, such as the consequences of: restrictions of advertising, fiscal controls, the differences between voluntary agreements and statutory mechanisms to regulate production, promotion and distribution, different types of crime prevention measures. A picture can be constructed of the gains and the losses – health, financial, and organizations – of each policy option for each participant in the policy process and the likely political will to change. Use of policy analysis can then be used to manipulate the consensual policy-making process. Organization networks may be manipulated by a number of persuasion techniques: information dissemination, incentives, and sanctions (Sharpe 1978). Such an approach need not opt simply for consensual, non-governmental, local policy preferences but might draw up a menu of policy options to be considered against overall objectives, whilst building up a knowledge of the network of organizations, alliances, and decisions that make up the complex policy environment. Only by thoroughly exploring the webs of decision making and the potential gains and losses to different parties can the potential for mutual adjustment be discovered.

In the study of healthy public policy on substance misuse, then, there exists differences in perspective, and the adoption of a particular approach has implications for the study and the development of policy. Adopting an out-and-out conflict perspective might run the risk of over-pessimism and a failure to make use of existing policy resources. On the other hand, the naive assumption of consensus could seriously underestimate the structural impediments to successful policy development. Each approach will favour a particular range of policy options. Conflict approaches are likely to favour state intervention to address issues of structural inequality. Consensual approaches are likely to stress more local non-state interventionist methods (though this is by no means universal). Clearly, no approach to policy development is without limitation and unintended consequence. Study of social policy and healthy public policy involves developing a reflexive awareness of the range of policy perspectives, within academic study and within the everyday policy environment.

CONCLUSION

Healthy public policy is fundamental to health promotion and is fast emerging as a discrete area of study. Conceived in very broad terms, it highlights many of the challenges encapsulated in Health For All 2000 and directs our attention to all aspects of the policy environment. Rhetoric on healthy public policy implies new ways of thinking about health and government policy and anticipates a new policy environment with new mechanisms for policy development. Such approaches might be seen to be commensurate with 'neo-liberal' government policy. In any case, understanding the existing policy environment is central to the development of healthy public policy. Such an understanding will draw upon a range of fields and disciplines, though social policy probably ranks as the nearest disciplinary ally. Any study of the policy context relating to health issues will necessarily draw upon the study of social policy.

A discipline itself fed by other disciplines, social policy comprises diverse perspectives. There are a number of perspectives on the appropriateness of state intervention. Differences in perspective depend upon basic assumptions about the nature of the social world. Healthy public policy can be seen to fall into similarly diverse perspectives. Substance misuse policy gives examples of clear differences amongst analysts – even though most will be working within a public health perspective. Conflict and consensus perspectives can be identified within this literature. Analysis of these perspectives provides understanding of the complexity of the study of, as well as the actual, social policy environment. Diversity in perspective is a feature of social policy and healthy public policy.

The study of social policy will contribute greatly to key areas of study within healthy public policy. These include understanding of: why healthy public policy features in today's policy environment, the role of the state, the citizen, and the community in policy development, the process and possibility of developing visions of healthy public policy, the scope for inter-sectoral co-operation, the scope for co-ordination of healthy public policy, and how the 'public good' might be reconciled with individual and other interests in fostering healthy public policy (Pederson *et al.* 1988). Such programmes of study are as pertinent to the development to social policy as they are to healthy public policy, making it feasible to consider health promotion as social policy.

REFERENCES

Ashton, J. and Seymour, H. (1988) *The New Public Health*, Milton Keynes: Open University Press.

Barrett, S. and Hill, M. J. (1984) 'Policy bargaining and structure in implementation of theory: towards an integrated perspective', *Policy and Politics* 12 (3): 219–40.

Beattie, A. (1991) 'Knowledge and control in health promotion: a test case for social policy and social theory', in J. Gabe, M. Calnan, and M. Bury (eds) *The Sociology of the Health Service*, London: Routledge.

Bell, D. (1960) *The End of Ideology*, New York: The Free Press.

Berridge, V. (1989) 'History and addiction control: the case of alcohol' in D. Robinson, A. Maynard, and R. Chester (eds) *Controlling Legal Addictions*, Basingstoke: Macmillan.

——(ed.) (1990) *Drug Research and Policy in Britain*, Aldershot: Avebury.

Beveridge, W. (1942) *Social Insurance and Allied Services*, Connol 6404, London: HMSO.

Blocker, J. S. (1976) *Retreat from Reform: The Prohibition Movement in the United States 1890–1913*, Westport, MA: Greenwood Press.

Blum, H. L. (1981) *Planning for Health: Genetics for the Eighties*, New York: Human Sciences Press.

Bocock, R., Clarke, J., Cochrane, A., Graham, P., and Wilson, M. (1987) *The State or the Market: Politics and Welfare in Contemporary Britain*, London: Sage in association with Open University Press.

Booth, M., Hartley, K., and Powell, M. (1990) 'Industry structure, performance and policy', in A. Maynard and P. Tether (eds) *Preventing Alcohol and Tobacco Problems*, Vol. 1, Aldershot: Avebury.

Booth, T. (1981a) 'Collaboration between the health and social services: part I, a case study in joint care planning?', *Policy and Politics* 9 (1): 23–49.

——(1981b) 'Collaboration between the health and social services: part II case study in joint finance', *Policy and Politics* 9 (2): 205–26.

Boulding, K. (1967) 'The boundaries of social policy', *Social Work* Vol 12 (1).

Brown, M. (1983) 'The development of social administration', in M. Loney, D. Boswell, and J. Clerke (eds) *Social Policy and Social Welfare*, Milton Keynes: Open University Press.

Bruce, M. (1961) *The Coming of the Welfare State*, London: Batsford.

Bruun, K. E. (1985) 'Formulating comprehensive national alcohol policies', in M. Grant (ed.) *Alcohol Policies*, European Series No 18, Copenhagen: WHO Regional Publications.

Bruun, K., Edwards, G., Lumio, M., Makela, K., Pan, L., Popham, R., Room, R., Schmidt, W., Skog, O., Sulkunen, P., and Osterberg, E. (1975) *Alcohol Control Policies in Public Health Perspective*, Finland: The Finnish Foundation for Alcohol Studies.

Bunton, R. (1990) 'Regulating our favourite Drug', in P. Abbott and G. Payne (eds) *New Directions in the Sociology of Health*, Basingstoke: Falmer.

Chapman-Walsh, D. (1990) 'The shifting boundaries of alcohol policy', *Health Affairs*, summer.

Crossland, C. A. R. (1956) *The Future of Socialism*, London: Cape.

Davies, P. and Walsh, D. (1983) *Alcohol Problems and Alcohol Control in Europe*, London: Croom Helm.

DHSS (1981) *Drinking Sensibly*, London: HMSO.

——(1989) *Interdepartmental Circular on Alcohol Misuse*, HN (89) 4 LAC (89) 6. WOC 8/89 WHC 89 (14).

Donati, P. (1988) 'The need for new social policy perspectives in health behaviour research', in R. Anderson, J. Davies, I. Kickbusch, D. McQueen, and D. Turner, (eds) *Health Behaviour Research and Health Promotion*, Oxford: Oxford University Press.

Donnison, D. (1979) 'Social policy since Titmuss', *Journal of Social Policy* 8 (2): 178–87.

Dorn, N. (1987) '*Drink and political economy*', in C. Heller *et al.* (eds) *Drug Use and Misuse: A Reader*, Chichester: Wiley in association with Open University.

Doyal, L. (1981) *The Political Economy of Health*, London: Pluto.

Duhl, L. J. (1986) *Health Planning and Social Change*, New York: Human Sciences Press.

Dye, R. R. (1976) *Policy Analysis*, Alabama: Alabama University Press.

Easton, D. (1953) *The Political System*, New York: Knopf.

Elston, M. A. (1991) 'The politics of professional power: medicine in a changing health service, in J. Gabe *et al.* (eds) *The Sociology of the Health Service*, London: Routledge.

Evers, A., Farrent, W., and Trojan, A. (eds) (1990) *Healthy Public Policy at the Local Level*, Colorado: Westview Press.

Farrent, W. and Taft, A. (1990) 'Building healthy public policy in an unhealthy climate: a case study from Paddington and North Kensington', in A. Evers, W. Farrent, and A. Trojan (eds) *Healthy Public Policy at the Local Level*, Colorado: Westview Press.

Fitzgerald, T. (1983) 'The new Right and the family', in M. Loney, D. Boswell, and J. Clark (eds) (1988) *Social Policy and Social Welfare*, Milton Keynes: Open University Press.

Freidson, E. (1970) *Profession of Medicine*, New York: Dodd, Mead.

Friedman, M. (1962) *Capitalism and Freedom*, Chicago: University of Chicago Press.

Furniss, N. and Tilton, T. (1977) *The Case for the Welfare State*, Indiana: Indiana University Press.

George, P. (1981) *Ideology and the Welfare State*, unpublished paper delivered to the Annual Conference of the Social Administration Association, Leeds University, July 1981.

George, P. and Manning, N. (1980) *Socialism, Social Welfare and the Soviet Union*, London: Routledge & Kegan Paul.

George, P. and Wilding, P. (1976) *Ideology and Social Welfare*, London: Routledge & Kegan Paul.

——(1985a) *Ideology and Social Welfare*, 2nd edn, London: Routledge & Kegan Paul.

——(1985b) *The Impact of Social Policy*, London: Routledge & Kegan Paul.

Gerhardt, V. (1989) *Ideas about Illness: An Intellectual and Political History of Medical Sociology*, London: Macmillan.

Godfrey, C. and Robinson, D. (eds) (1990) *Preventing Alcohol and Tobacco Problems*, vol. 2, Aldershot: Avebury.

Gordon, I., Lewis, J. and Young, K. (1977) 'Perspectives on policy analysis', *Public Administration Bulletin* 25.

Grant, M. (1985) (eds) *Alcohol Policies*, European Series No 18, Geneva: WHO Regional Publications.

——(1989) 'Controlling alcohol abuse', in D. Robinson, A. Maynard, and R. Chester (eds) *Controlling Legal Addictions*, Basingstoke: Macmillan.

Gray, H. and Sheldon, A. (1969) *Universal and Selective Social Benefits*, London: Institute of Economic Affairs.

Gusfield, J. R. (1963) *Symbolic Crusade*, Urbana: University of Illinois Press.

Ham, C. and Hill, C. (1984) *The Policy Process in the Modern Capitalist State*, Brighton: Wheatsheaf Books.

Hannock, T. (1982) 'Beyond health care', *The Futurist*, August: 4–13.

Harrison, B. (1971) *Drink and the Victorians: The Temperance Question in England, 1815–1872*, London: Faber.

Harrison, L. and Tether, P. (1990) 'Tax policy: structure and process', in A. Maynard and D. Tether (eds) *Preventing Alcohol and Tobacco Problems*, vol. 1, Aldershot: Avebury.

Hartnoll, R. (1989) 'The international context', in S. MacGregor (ed.) *Drugs and British Society: Responses to a Social Problem in the 1980s*, London: Routledge.

Hawks, D. V. (1990) 'The watering down of Australia's health policy on alcohol', *Drug and Alcohol Review* 9 (1): 91–5.

Heller, T., Gott, M., and Jeffery, C. (eds) (1987) *Drug Use and Misuse: A Reader*, Chichester: Wiley in association with the Open University.

Hogwood, B. W. and Gunn, L. A. (1981) *The Policy Orientation*, Strathclyde: Centre for the Study of Public Policy, University of Strathclyde.

Home Office (1987a) *Young People and Alcohol: Report of the Working Group of the Standing Conference on Crime Prevention*, London: Home Office.

——(1987b) *The Licensing Act 1964 Government Proposals for Reforms*, London: Home Office.

Jacobson, B. (1981) *The Lady Killers*, London: Pluto.

Jones, K. (1954) *Lunacy, Law and Conscience* London: Routledge & Kegan Paul.

Kendell, R. E. (1987) 'Drinking sensibly; the first Benno Pollak Lecture', *British Journal of Addiction* 82: 1279–88.

Koskikallio, I. (1979) 'Socio-economic functions of Finish restaurants', *British Journal of Addiction* 74: 67–78.

Lee, P. and Raban, C. (1983) 'Welfare and ideology', in M. Loney, D. Boswell, and J. Clerke (eds) (1988) *Social Policy and Social Welfare*, Milton Keynes: Open University Press.

Legg, D. and Sylvan, L. (1990) 'Community participation in health: the Consumers' Health Forum and the Victoria District Health Council Programme', in A.G. Evers, W. Farrent, and A. Trojan (eds) *Healthy Public Policy at the Local Level*, Colorado: Westview Press.

Le Grand, J. (1982) *The Strategy of Equality*, London: Allen & Unwin.

Levine, H. G. (1978) 'The discovery of addiction: changing conceptions of habitual drunkenness in America', *Journal of Studies on Alcohol* 39: 143–74.

Lindblorn, C. (1965) *The Intelligence of Democracy*, New York: The Free Press.

Loney, M. (ed.) (1987) *The State or the Market*, London: Sage.

Loney, M., Boswell, D. and Clerke, J. (eds) (1988) *Social Policy and Social Welfare*, Milton Keynes: Open University Press.

MacGregor, S. (eds) (1989) *Drugs and British Society: Responses to a Social Problem in the 1980s*, London: Routledge.

Makela, K. and Viikari, M. (1977) 'Notes on alcohol and the state', *Acta Sociologica* 20: 155–79.

Makela, K., Room, R., Single, E., Sulkunen, P., and Walsh, B. (1981) *Alcohol, Society and the State*, Vol. 1, Toronto: Addiction Research Foundation.

Manning, N. (1985) 'Constructing social problems', in N. Manning (ed.) *Social Problems and Welfare Ideology*, Aldershot: Gower.

Marshall, T. H. (1975) *Social Policy*, 4th edition, London: Hutchinson.

Marshall, T. H. and Rees, A. M. (1985) *T. H. Marshall's Social Policy*, London: Hutchinson.

Maynard, A. and Robinson, D. (1990) 'Preventing Alcohol and Tobacco Problems', in Godfrey, C. and Robinson, D. (eds) *Preventing Alcohol and Tobacco Problems* Vol. 2; Aldershot: Avebury.

Maynard, A. and Tether, P. (eds) (1990) *Preventing Alcohol and Tobacco Problems*, Vol. 1 Aldershot: Avebury.

Milio, N. (1986) *Promoting Health Through Public Policy*, Ottawa: Canadian Public Health Association.

——(1987) *Healthy Public Policy: Issues and Scenarios*, unpublished paper prepared for a Symposium on Healthy Public Policy, Yale University, 5 October 1987.

Mishra, R. (1977) *Society and Social Policy*, London: Macmillan.

——(1984) *The Welfare State in Crisis*, London: Wheatsheaf.

Navarro, V. (1976) *Medicine Under Capitalism*, London: Croom Helm.

——(1982) 'The crisis of the international capitalist order and its implications for the welfare state', *International Journal of Health Services* 12 (2): 169–90.

——(1986) *Crisis, Health and Medicine: A Social Critique*, London: Tavistock.

Ottawa Charter (1986) *The Ottawa Charter for Health Promotion*, WHO: Health and Welfare Canada and Canadian Public Health Association.

Parker, D. (1977) 'Alcohol control policy and the fiscal crisis of the state', *Drinking and Drug Practices Survey* 13 (December): 3–6.

Pascall, G. (1986) *Social Policy: A Feminist Analysis*, London: Tavistock.

Pederson, A. P., Edwards, R. K., Kelner, M., Marshall, V. W., and Allison, K. R. (1988) 'Coordinating healthy public policy: an analytic literature review and bibliography', *Health Services and Promotion Branch Working Paper HSPB 88–1*, Toronto: Health and Welfare Canada.

Pinker, R. (1979) *The Idea of Welfare*, London: Heinemann.

Redding, M. (1970) 'Universality and selectivity', in W. Robson and B. Crick (eds) *The Future of Social Services*, Harmondsworth: Penguin.

Rein, M. (1970) *Social Policy: Issues of Choice and Change*, London: Random House.

Rex, J. (1978) 'British sociology's war of religion', *New Society*, 11 May.

Robinson, D. (1989) 'Controlling legal addictions: "taking advantage of what's there"', in D. Robinson, A. Maynard, and R. Chester (eds) *Controlling Legal Addictions*, Basingstoke: Macmillan.

Robinson, D. and Maynard, A. (1990) 'Preventing alcohol and tobacco problems', in C. Godfrey and C. Robinson (eds) *Preventing Alcohol and Tobacco Problems*, Vol. 2, Aldershot: Avebury.

Robinson, D., Maynard, A., and Chester, R. (1989) *Controlling Legal Addictions*, Basingstoke: Macmillan.

Robinson, D., Tether, P., and Teller, J. (1989) *Preventing Alcohol Problems: A Guide for Local Action*, London: Tavistock.

Rodgers, B. N. *et al.* (1968) *Comparative Social Administration*, London: Allen & Unwin.

Room, G. (1979) *The Sociology of Welfare*, London: Blackwell.

Room, R. (1981) 'The case for a problem prevention approach to alcohol, drug and mental problems', *Public Health Reports* 96: 26–33.

Royal College of Physicians (1987) *A Great and Growing Evil*, London: Tavistock.

Sabatier, P. A. (1986) 'Top-down and bottom-up approaches to implementation research: a critical analysis and suggested synthesis', *Journal of Public Policy* 6 (1): 21–48.

Senoda, K. (1990) 'Health promotion and consumers' cooperative movements in Japan', in A. Evers, W. Farrent, and A. Trojan (eds) *Healthy Public Policy at the local level*, Colorado: Westview Press.

Sharpe, L. J. (1978) 'The social scientist and policy making in Britain and America: a comparison', in M. Bulmer (ed.) Social Policy Research, London: Macmillan.

Small, N. (1988) 'AIDS and social policy', *Critical Social Policy* 21 (Spring): 9–29.

Stacey, M. (1988) 'Strengthening communities', *International Conference on Health Promotion, Ottawa, Canada: Selected Conference Proceedings*, Ottawa: WHO, Health and Welfare Canada, and Canadian Public Health Association.

Stimson, G. (1987) 'British drug policies in the 1980s: a preliminary analysis and suggestions for research', *British Journal of Addiction* 82: 477.

Strong, P. M. (1986) 'A new modelling of medicine? Comments on the WHO's regional strategy for Europe', *Social Science and Medicine* 22 (2): 193–9.

Sulkunen, P. (1985) 'International aspects of the prevention of alcohol problems: research experiences and perspectives', in M. Grant (ed.) *Alcohol Policies*, Copenhagen: WHO.

Taylor, P. (1984) *Smoking Ring*, London: Bodley Head.

Tether, P. and Robinson, D. (1986) *Preventing Alcohol Problems: A Guide for Local Action*, London: Tavistock.

Titmuss, R. M. (1968) 'Address to the Social Administration Association', quoted in M. Brown (1983).

——(1968) *Commitment to Welfare*, London: Allen & Unwin.

——(1974) *Social Policy*, London: Allen & Unwin.

Townsend, P. (ed.) (1968) *Social Services for All?*, London: Fabian Society.

——(ed.) (1975) *Sociology and Social Policy*, London: Allen & Unwin.

Van der Kamp, J. (1990) 'Managing health promotion as an open process: holistic and ecological tools for managing and marketing of innovations', in A. Evers, W. Farrent, and A. Trojan (eds) *Healthy Public Policy at a Local Level*, Colorado: Westview.

Van Lennep, E. (1980) 'From the welfare state to the welfare society' *OECD Observer* 107: 19–20.

Waitzkin, H. (1983) *The Second Sickness: Contradictions of Capitalist Health Care*, New York: Free Press.

Waitzkin, H. and Waterman, B. (1974) *The Exploitation of Illness in Capitalist Society*, New York: Bobbs-Merrill.

Walker, A. (1983) 'Social policy, social administration and the social construction of welfare', in M. Loney, D. Boswell, and J. Clerke (eds) *Social Policy and Social Welfare*, Milton Keynes: Open University Press.

Walsh, B. and Grant, M. (1985) *Public Health Implications of Alcohol Production and Trade*, Geneva: WHO.

Widavsky, A. (1979) *Speaking Truth To Power: The Art and Craft of Policy Analysis*, Boston: Little Brown.

Wilding, P. (1982) *Professional Power and Social Welfare*, London: Routledge & Kegan Paul.

——(ed.) (1986) *In Defence of the Welfare State*, Manchester: Manchester University Press.

Wilson, E. (1983) 'Feminism and social policy', in M. Loney, D. Boswell, and J. Clerke (eds) *Social Policy and Social Welfare*, Milton Keynes: Open University Press.

Wittrock, R. and De Leon, P. (1986) 'Policy as a moving target: a call for conceptual realism', *Policy Studies Review* 6 (1): 44–60.

WHO (1985) *Targets for Health For All*, Copenhagen: WHO Regional Office for Europe.

——(1986) *Intersectoral Action for Health; the Role of Intersectoral Cooperation in National Strategies for Health For All*, Geneva: WHO.

——(1988a) *Health Policies to Combat Drug and Alcohol Problems*, A Satellite Conference to the Healthy Public Policy Conference, Sydney and Canberra, Australia, 24–31 March 1988. Consensus Statement prepared by WHO Expert Working Group, Geneva: WHO.

——(1988b) *The Adelaide Recommendations, Healthy Public Policy*, Copenhagen: WHO/EURO.

Ziglio, E. (1987) 'Policy making and planning in conditions of uncertainty: theoretical considerations for health promotion policy', *Draft Working Paper No 7*, Edinburgh: Research Unit in Health and Behavioural Change.

Chapter 8

Social marketing and health promotion

Craig Lefebvre

Social marketing is an orientation to health promotion in which programmes are developed to satisfy consumers needs, strategized to reach the audience(s) in need of the programme, and managed to meet organizational objectives (Lefebvre and Flora 1988). It is a set of principles and techniques that derive from a theoretical perspective based in marketing as it has been developed and practised in the business sector; however, social marketing practitioners borrow heavily from other disciplines (many of them reviewed in other chapters of this book) in conceptualizing approaches to changing people's attitudes and behaviours.

In one respect, social marketing has existed as long as people have sought to 'win people's hearts and minds'. Social marketing is concerned with introducing and disseminating new ideas and issues (Fine 1981) and increasing the prevalence of specific behaviours among target groups. Thus, when we examine major religious and political leaders, artists and scholars, social advocates and philosophers over the years, we are looking at people who were, at one level or another, social marketers. The extent to which these people are known to us, the impact their lives had in their own time, as well as now, and the endurance of their ideas reflect as much their success – or that of their followers – to 'market' the ideas as they do their creativity, intellect, and influence on improving people's lives. However, the term 'social marketing' was formally coined by Kotler and Zaltman (1971) to define a process in which marketing techniques and concepts are applied to social issues and causes instead of products and services.

Social marketing has evolved from business practices in which a 'product' and 'sales' orientation have been supplanted by a 'consumer' one. That is, businesses are now more likely to focus on consumers' wants and needs and trying to meet them than they are on simply producing whatever they like and then trying to convince consumers to buy it. In health promotion the parallel process has been from a more traditional 'top-down' approach in which authorities prescribe, or proscribe, health and social behaviours, and perhaps launch information campaigns to support the programmes, to 'bottom-up' efforts where the needs and wants of the people are actively solicited, attended to, and acted upon in programme planning, delivery, management, and evaluation. At its most simple, social marketing is a consumer-orientated approach that creates 'win-win' situations for all parties. Yet, as this chapter will illustrate, it is a very systematic approach to health and social issues that is limited only by the imagination of the social marketing programme.

With this overview of social marketing, it is also important to state what it is not. Social marketing is not social control; it is not focused only on changing individuals' beliefs, attitudes, and behaviours; it is not simply mass media campaigns; and it is not easy. Social marketing is a method of empowering people to be totally involved and responsible for their well-being; a problem-solving process that may suggest new and innovative ways to attack health and social problems (e.g. Manoff 1985; Novelli 1984); it is a comprehensive strategy for effecting social change on a broad scale (Lefebvre and Flora 1988); and it requires careful planning, research, and management to implement effectively.

This chapter begins with a review of the eight essential characteristics of a social marketing approach as outlined by Lefebvre and Flora (1988). This will lead to a discussion of the challenges that are posed to social marketers – especially the lack of adequate research to support social marketing's utility and effectiveness. Finally, we will conclude with a review of the field and a focus on the benefits social marketing offers health promotion endeavours.

CHARACTERISTICS OF SOCIAL MARKETING

Lefebvre and Flora (1988) propose eight characteristics of social marketing programmes; they are listed in Table 8.1. These components are not

Table 8.1 Social marketing components

Consumer orientation
Exchange theory
Audience segmentation and analysis
Formative research
Channel analysis
Marketing mix
Message/product/service
Price
Place
Promotion
Positioning
Process tracking
Management system

Source: Lefebvre and Flora 1988

necessarily displayed by every programme professing to be a social market-ing' one, yet the authors stress their importance in the analysis, implemen-tation, management, and evaluation of public health programmes. The next sections describe each component in some detail.

Consumer orientation

At the heart of a marketing approach are the consumers one wishes to reach and influence. Two approaches to these consumers are possible. An agency can conceive of its target audience as essentially passive and seek to understand their wants and needs in a context of 'doing something for them'. Such an orientation will often lead to a series of messages/products/services that are designed to meet these needs, but have little direct input from consumers themselves. One weakness of this approach, as will be shown later, is that while great care is given to audience segmentation and analysis, the formative research process is forsaken. A second limitation of this approach to the consumer is most apparent when social marketing programmes are applied in a community organization context. Here we find that the crucial community organization principle of citizen participation in all aspects of programme planning, delivery, and evaluation is sacrificed as well. While many social marketing programmes have met their short-term objectives of changing people's awareness, knowledge, and behaviour, these same programmes often do not address the social and institutional contours that influence individual behaviours nor do they have the community support needed to sustain them over the longer term when external funding cycles are completed (cf. Lefebvre 1990).

The second approach to the consumer is an active one; that is, assuming that consumer input to the proposed programme is a continuing process and not one that occurs at a single point in time. The emphasis of this approach to consumers is to seek to build relationships with them over time and continually offer them opportunities to interact with programme staff. In one variant of this type of approach, lay people from the community become integral parts of the programme and assist in the actual implementation next to the professional staff (Lefebvre *et al.* 1986). Such a structure allows for dialogue between staff and community resident on a daily basis. These volunteers become the representatives of the larger set of 'consumers', and can provide the immediate feedback to staff as to how proposed programmes will be accepted by the community. They can also act as the sentinels for programmes that may not be appropriate to the community, or specific segments of it, because of social, cultural, and political norms not apparent to programme planners.

A consumer orientation does not mean that all health promotion pro-grammes must be grassroots efforts that only build from citizens' concerns.

Many health programmes are launched because of epidemiological data gathered by health authorities that identify health problems of sufficient magnitude to warrant attention. In many cases, citizens may not be aware of the scope of a health problem or health risk that has been identified. Consequently, a first priority of an information campaign is to alert the public to the problem. However, it is often the next step, engaging people into the process, that is overlooked by the planners of these programmes. Citizen participation at this stage can lay the foundation for community ownership of the effort and sculpt the next phases of the programme. It is the types of programmes that do not enlist community involvement that are decried as 'experiments in social control'. For health promotion efforts in the coming decades, it is clear that the consumer (read the 'community') must be treated as, and encouraged to be, an active partner in the process.

An orientation that favours the primacy of the consumer is intuitively and philosophically appealing to health promotion professionals; yet there are barriers to them, and their organizations, immediately and wholeheartedly embracing it. Among these barriers are (1) a failure by the organization to define its mission and objectives clearly due to a lack of inter-organizational consensus and inadequate consumer assessment; (2) not identifying key target audiences which results in a lack of focus and poorly targeted needs surveys; (3) pressures that place political/territorial/professional objectives above consumer needs; (4) organizational biases that favour expert-driven programmes; (5) the influence of intermediaries who modify the programmes' messages, products, and services before they reach the target group; and (6) the sense of urgency that often accompanies new initiatives and provides a rationalization for 'short cuts' (cf. Lefebvre and Flora 1988). It is this latter point that especially requires more attention from programme planners and policy makers. Too often it is our search for the 'quick fix' or the imposition of short timelines that leads to inadequate attention to the target group. While this is not to suggest that planning should be a protracted process, time needs to be allocated to secure proper needs assessments and community participation prior to programme implementation.

An orientation to health promotion that has the consumer public at its nexus must not only focus on consumers' wants and needs prior to programme implementation, but has to consider the satisfaction of consumers with the programme after its delivery. Satisfying consumer needs is the major objective of a marketing approach; evaluations of marketing programmes should reflect these issues as much as the 'objective' or 'hard' data of behaviour and physiological change.

Exchange theory

The operational mechanism for marketing practices of all kinds is exchange theory (Kotler 1975). Whether it be an idea, a product, or a service, the offering by one agent (i.e. an individual, group, or organization) is done within a context where the other agent has the choice to 'buy' it or not. Thus, marketing is the voluntary exchange of resources between two or more parties, and includes processes of information dissemination, public relations, lobbying, advocacy, and fund raising (Fine 1981). In social marketing, the resources we seek to exchange with our target audience are usually different from the more common form of exchanges in which money is offered for goods and services (though by no means does this exclude such transactions in a social marketing programme). Rather, social marketing is the exchange of an intangible for an intangible: accepting a new idea and discarding an old custom or adopting a new behaviour and giving up a habit. It is not easy, nor desirable, to try and give monetary value to these types of transactions. However, social marketers must recognize that different economies still come into play as a consumer weighs the costs and benefits of, for example, quitting smoking or using condoms. Consumers pay a price in terms of the time it takes to learn new information or practice new behaviours; they expend cognitive and physical effort; they risk alienating family members and friends when adopting new ideas and practices; and they may be perceived by the community-at-large as being 'different'. Public health agencies, on the other hand, often do not assess their resources appropriately to facilitate such exchanges. Whether it be their financial resources, technical expertise, their ideas, products, or services, these agencies often underestimate their value. The tendency to 'give it away' needs to be examined. The image of a consumer saying 'Why should I if they don't think it's that valuable?' has to be addressed by social marketers before the question is actually asked.

Social marketing involves consumers exchanging resources for new beliefs and behaviours. It is not a simple task to define this exchange tangibly, but it often does not need to be done. Many social marketing programmes become so focused on 'making the intangible tangible' through product and service development coupled with strong advertising campaigns that it is often overlooked that exchanges can still be effected in the cognitive domain alone. The strategy is to create an awareness among consumers that they have a problem and then offer the solution. Commercial marketers have long employed this strategy as they successfully sell everything from soap to deodorants to automobiles. The problem may relate to possible social disapproval or to lowered self-esteem. It may also appeal to more positive benefits such as greater self-confidence and success.

Social marketers sometimes offer solutions to problems that are not well defined for the average consumer. Marketers can take for granted that people are aware of the prevalence and lethality of certain health risks and pose new information and behavioural prescriptions without answering the consumer's basic question: 'What's the benefit to me?'. While costs often become the marketers' prime concern in developing a programme it may be the other side of the equation – the benefits – that are of at least equal importance to the consumer. Most consumer behaviour theory suggests that it is the relative balance of costs *and* benefits that leads a consumer to accept a new idea, behaviour, product, or service. While it is important to reduce costs to the consumer to make health accessible to them, it is the perceived benefits that will determine consumer's motivation to access these resources and change. As noted earlier, it is maximizing these benefits, and communicating them clearly to consumers in ways that are meaningful to them, that distinguishes good social marketing practice. Well-crafted marketing programmes meet both consumer needs and organizational objectives (win-win).

Audience segmentation and analysis

Social marketing requires knowledge of target groups, including their sociodemographic, psychological, and behavioural characteristics (Kotler and Roberto 1989). Social marketers may aim at changing attitudes and behaviours of the public-at-large, but they approach this task by selecting and targeting subgroups of this larger population that are homogeneous with respect to one or more characteristics (e.g. lower-class minority males, middle-aged males who are contemplating becoming more physically active, the food buyer for a family). It is the process of identifying and researching these segments that is the foundation, the nucleus of programme development.

Weinstein (1987) has identified four major benefits of audience segmentation and analysis. First, by understanding the unique needs of target groups, messages, products, and services can be developed that meet the needs of those groups; this reinforces the consumer orientation and enhances the prospect of meeting organizational objectives. Segmentation also helps one determine the most cost-efficient ways to promote messages/products/services to target groups. Segmentation can also place one's programming efforts in relation to other ideas, preferences, or behaviours already held or practised by the target group (the notion of 'positioning'). Finally, segmentation allows for a systematic approach to market coverage, rather than relying on a 'shot-gun' approach to mass marketing in which many groups, often those most in most need of the message, are missed.

In developing a segmentation analysis, one must have homogeneity within each segment and heterogeneity between segments on the variable(s) of interest (Weinstein 1987; Fine 1981). Segments should also be of sufficient size to warrant the allocation of organizational resources; should be relevant and meaningful for the message, product, or service to be delivered; and should suggest different marketing mixes for each segment (Weinstein 1987; Fine 1981). However, the actual approach to segmenting a population will be based on organizational objectives, theoretical tenets, and past research and experience. There is no 'right' or 'wrong' approach to segmentation as long as formative research is undertaken to assure the match of theory and experience with present realities. Some variables along which market segmentation may be conducted are shown in Table 8.2.

Table 8.2   Market segmentation variables

Sociodemographic variables	Behavioural	Psychological
Location (community, neighbourhood)	Use of product/service	Self-esteem
	Benefits sought	Readiness for change
Household size	Level of physical activity	Introspective
Age	Use of leisure time	Sensation seeker
Sex	Level of sexual activity	Hedonism
Race	Health professional	Achievement orientated
Nationality	utilization pattern	Need for independence
Religion		Societally conscious
Marital status		Belongers
Education		Need for approval
Occupation		Need for power
Income		
Social class		

Market segmentation does not need to be confined to individuals; social systems are also segmentation candidates as well. Social systems are easily divided into sector 'segments' – educational, industry, government, health, etc. These sectors can be further segmented by location (e.g. urban vs. rural health departments), membership size of composite units (e.g. larger school districts vs. smaller ones), type of business (e.g. service industries vs. manufacturing vs. agricultural), current practices (e.g. businesses with active health promotion programmes for employees), organizational factors (e.g. innovativeness, leadership style, employee participation, community involvement), characteristics associated with organizational innovativeness (e.g. centralization, complexity, formalization, interconnectedness, organizational slack, size; Rogers 1983), and many other variables. In developing broad-based health promotion programmes, attention to organizational segmentation is as necessary as population segmentation techniques in crafting comprehensive intervention strategies.

Formative research

Formative research is used here to denote research activities conducted prior to full implementation of a social marketing strategy. Indeed, formative research is best utilized when it contributes to the development of the strategy itself. These research activities include studies of audience segment needs and characteristics, market analyses to determine positioning strategies, pretesting of concepts and messages, and pilot tests of message/product/service acceptability and effectiveness. There are numerous methodologies that the social marketer can employ in designing formative studies including traditional surveys, randomized designs, panel studies, focus groups, convenience samples, 'snowball' sampling (in which early participants suggest others 'like them' for subsequent contact), piggybacking on studies being conducted by other organizations, and reviews of secondary data sources – such as research studies published in scientific and marketing journals, government and private sector reports, marketing studies sponsored by industry, and epidemiological surveys.

Kotler and Andreasen (1987) underscore the importance of engaging in more, not less, market research, and identify five 'myths' that appear to dampen enthusiasm for research activities among the not-for-profit sector. These myths are:

1 The 'big decision' myth in which only projects that involve large investments of money and/or staff time are deemed suitable for research effort. However, the costs of conducting a research project – in terms of monetary investment, time needed to complete it, delays in decision making – should be analysed in comparison to its potential benefits – improvements in decision making from more information, avoiding 'square wheels', possibly suggesting new ideas or solutions. Not all formative research involves time-consuming and expensive organizational outlays. Qualitative methods such as focus groups and consumer panels can be quite efficient in providing programme managers a better sense of consumer response than simply going with the 'best idea'.

2 The 'survey myopia' myth is related to the last comment. Market research does not need to consist of only random surveys of target groups with their expenses related to design, conduct, data management, analysis, interpretation, and report preparation – let alone time. Limited and modest research objectives can be met by modest and inexpensive research strategies. The key is to elucidate clearly the objective of the research and interpret the data in the context in which it was collected.

3 The 'big bucks' myth also builds on the first two myths: however, research has lower cost alternatives. While there is certainly a sacrifice of one's ability to generalize from qualitative research methods, in many

instances the marketer's objective is to 'get a feel' for the target group, not to draw scientifically valid conclusions for the general population.

4 The 'sophisticated researcher' myth obscures the notion that organizations do not require staff with expertise in sampling design and statistical analyses in order to undertake a valuable market research programme. What is needed are (a) clear objectives (questions), (b) a strategy that will elicit responses from the target group's representatives (however selected) in a consistent manner, (c) objective documentation of respondents' answers and comments (i.e. audio recordings of focus groups rather than a facilitator's overall conclusions; questionnaires that are administered and tallied consistently across respondents), (d) staff and other organizational resource allocations to fully implement the research protocol, and (e) timely feedback of useful information to project managers.

5 The 'most research is not read' myth reflects as much a manager's lack of interest in, or even fear of, research results as it does the fact that researchers and programme managers often do not communicate well in identifying the decision that requires additional information and how the information needs to be collected and analysed in order to be useful to decision makers. These points reinforce the observation that managers who are not consumer orientated, but would rather follow their own preconceived ideas, will not support market research. However, it is also the case that unless 'implementors' and 'evaluators' are working together in designing research protocols, the best intentions may go for nought.

Even if the only market research an organization does is to challenge each staff member to talk with ten representatives from a target group every week, the ability to stay in close touch with consumers is too important simply to take for granted once the initial 'problem identification' stage of programme planning is completed. For social marketing programmes to be effective, and stay effective over the long term, a commitment to an on-going market research programme is vital.

Channel analysis

Channel analysis is the specification and understanding of communication and distribution systems as they relate to discrete target groups. Although channel analysis could be considered part of audience analysis and formative research – especially as it relates to identifying appropriate channels through which to reach target populations – it has been separated out here both to reinforce its importance in marketing programmes and also to underscore that channels of message, product, and service distribution are critical to successful programmes.

In their analysis of what constitutes a successful public information campaign, Rice and Atkin (1989) elucidate several components directly relevant to channels:

1 It is necessary to identify and understand the media habits of the target groups.
2 Characteristics of the message source and its media help determine a campaign's effectiveness.
3 The message must reach a sufficiently large proportion of the target population in order for the campaign to be successful in meeting its objectives.
4 Messages must go through multiple channels to ensure their accessibility and appropriateness to the target group.

Lefebvre and Flora (1988) presented several more components of media that need to be considered and explored in channel analysis:

1 Their relative abilities to transmit complex messages.
2 Whether the medium is electronic or print, visual or auditory (or both), and how that will affect message design and delivery as well as audience attention, comprehension, and retention.
3 Their relative costs given their expected reach and impact.
4 Their reach, frequency of message delivery, and the continuity that can be created and controlled by the sponsoring organization.
5 The number of intermediaries that the media require – the more intermediaries involved, typically the less control one has over final message structure and content.
6 Each medium's potential for overuse both in terms of oversaturating a market to the extent that the target group 'turns off' the message and becomes inattentive, and the degree to which excessive demands are made on media gatekeepers which then turns them against the organization and future collaborative projects.
7 Each medium's capability to build on, or multiply, the effects achieved through another medium.

In analysing channels, one assumption that is often made by social marketing programmes is to treat channels as if communication of messages is the primary objective. Some authors assert that message design and dissemination are the major tasks of a social marketing programme (Manoff 1985). In many cases this may not be the case. While message delivery may be an important aspect of health promotion, distribution of related products and services is often what achieves the desired results, yet this aspect of channel analysis usually receives little attention. For example, in the DuaLima test market study (Doremus Porter Novelli 1986), many questions about the contraceptive marketing programme revolved around more distribution-driven concerns such as 'What type of retail outlets should be used in getting a new product into the consumer market-place?' 'What margin is required to interest the retail trade in selling the brand (of contraceptive)?' Some of these issues relate to 'Place' decisions as part of the marketing mix; yet, sufficient information needs to be gathered early on in the developmental process to permit better decision making.

The marketing mix

The marketing mix refers to what are historically the four pillars of marketing programmes – the '4 Ps': product, place, price, and promotion. The 'mix' of these four elements to meet the needs of specific market segments is the operationalization of the marketing concept. While the '4 Ps' have carried marketers far in planning and implementing effective campaigns, in today's more competitive market-place (not just for products and services, but ideas as well) one must also incorporate a fifth 'P' into the mix: position. The next sections review each element of the marketing mix.

Product

Fine (1981) provides a useful definition of 'product' as it may be expressed in social marketing programmes: 'anything having the ability to satisfy human needs or wants'. He also points out that the true test of whether this 'thing' is, or is not, a product also rests on its capacity for exchangeability; simply, are people willing to trade for it (i.e. pay a 'price')? Three types of products can thus be defined for social marketers. The first, messages, or the communication of information intended to influence the receiver's attention, knowledge, motivation, and/or behaviour (McGuire 1984), are the most common type of social marketing programme. The dissemination of 'information products' comprises the major thrust of public information, or health communication, campaigns. The creation of messages that are both scientifically sound in content and possess the creative ability to capture attention and reliably communicate the content to the desired audience are necessary features of social marketing programmes. However, it is often the tension between 'science' and 'art' (the content vs. the execution strategy) that leads to less than effective message design. Most health programmes appear to favour 'science' over 'art': what this results in are scientifically sound messages that are so dense, long-winded, presented at too high a literacy level, and in styles and layouts not conducive to attention or retention, that their impact on the target group is negligible. However, this is not meant to suggest 'glitz' over substance; rather, the dynamism should result in more creative work where art is employed to present the science. Independent of the scientific content, there are other features of message design that will affect the attention, comprehension, and retention processes of the receiver. Table 8.3 presents a list of content, design, persuasion, and memorability factors identified by Manoff (1985).

Table 8.3   Factors affecting message design strategy

Content	Persuasion	Design	Memorability
The problem	Reason why	The single idea	Idea reinforcement
Target audience	Empathy	Language and cultural	Minimizing distractions
Resistance points	Concern arousal	relevance	Reprise (repetition)
Solution	Action capability	Situation and character	
Required action	Believability	identification	
Authoritative source	Creativity	Distinctive message style	
	Benefits	Low fatigue index	

Source: Manoff 1985: 197–203

It is also important to note that message dissemination in and of itself may not be sufficient to meet consumer needs or organizational objectives. Message support through the addition of 'tangible' products and services may also be required to reinforce and amplify critical features of the message that do not lend themselves to mediated activities. For instance, support groups for persons with HIV infection or video products to use for exercising at home.

Tangible products that can be used by consumers is the second product category. These products might range from condoms in family planning projects to school curricula for AIDS education to self-help materials for smoking cessation in various formats (print, electronic, video). An even broader view of products was taken by Lefebvre and Flora (1988) who characterized any tangible representation of an agency to its markets as a product; this definition would encompass posters, brochure, and other message media from which consumers might draw certain conclusions about the organization. Such an approach to products leads an agency to adopt very specific guidelines about the development of materials, including size, colour, and location of programme logotypes; uniformity in layout; and specific language to describe the organizational mission, sponsoring agencies, and similar content features. The goal of such efforts is to establish a consistent approach to the consumer market one is targeting so that programme identity is established and reinforced on each consumer exposure to the organization. This is in contrast to a less formalized approach wherein each brochure an organization puts out has a different 'look and feel' to it, rendering it much more difficult to position the organization to its market. Success (and sometimes failure!) in these efforts is seen when quick glimpses of, or short phrases from, these materials result in correct identification by consumers of the originating agency ('It looks like something from the XYZ department!').

Products have a number of properties that should be addressed in the formative stages. Among the more important attributes of products to consider are brand name (title), features (e.g. ease of use, self-directed instruction), styling and packaging (an 'upmarket' appearance, a traditional cultural appeal), colour, and size. Other more subjective product attributes from a consumer's point of view might include: efficacy, expected benefit, safety, fit with current lifestyle, possibility of trial usage, and relative value to current product usage (or non-usage).

Many health promotion programmes feature service delivery as the cornerstone of their change efforts. In the large US community heart disease prevention studies, service delivery of one type or another was deemed essential to facilitating the individual change process. Such service delivery included screening, counselling, and referral events; adult education groups on topics of nutrition, smoking cessation, and exercise; worksite health promotion consultation and programmes; and work with food retailers to implement point-of-purchase nutrition education programmes. Clearly, many other programme components fit the service mode, including hotlines, self-help groups, consultation work, individual and family counselling, and social welfare assistance. Service delivery is often the method by which organizations structure their direct, face-to-face contacts with target markets (or clients). These interpersonal encounters are found to be the most important factor in producing changes in behaviour of the target group (Rice and Atkin 1989; Rogers 1983).

The creation of services usually arises from identified needs of specific populations and is developed from any one of a variety of philosophical and theoretical perspectives. It is not the intent here to outline the 'best' way to develop services; it is sufficient here to reiterate that such services should have a consumer-driven rationale and that formative studies document their efficacy in addressing the problem. The marketing of services, once developed and tested, does offer some unique problems to be considered.

Kotler and Bloom (1984) describe several challenges unique to service marketing. These challenges include:

> Service marketers must be as attentive to 'third parties' as they are to primary target groups. Health professionals have certain ethical and practice norms that directly impact on what they can, and cannot do, in response to 'patient demand'. Government agencies and insurance companies are other 'silent' consumers who may not be directly involved in consumer-provider exchanges, but their influence does indirectly affect such factors as the scope, content, outcome, and even availability of some services.

> Services are by their very nature less capable of being evaluated by consumers before, and many times after, being used. For example, it is difficult for clients to compare rival smoking cessation programmes and assess whether the chosen programme really did reduce the chance of developing lung cancer. Thus, client education becomes an even more important issue to address when marketing services.

Maintaining high levels of quality control becomes a core function, especially as the number of people engaging in the delivery of the service increases. Staff training and supervision require on-going organizational commitments of time and effort. The varying backgrounds of people involved in health promotion service delivery – ranging from physicians to community nurses to dietitians to lay volunteers – makes this an area particularly vulnerable to undermining if proper acknowledgement and care is not given to quality control audits and monitoring.

Many professionals involved in service delivery have neither the knowledge, experience, time, and/or inclination to undertake marketing activities. Hopefully, as more is learned about successful marketing practice in the service sector, and health professionals shed their reluctance to become health marketers, we will witness a changing practice pattern in which ethical and socially responsible marketing practice enhances the delivery and efficacy of health services to the public.

Price

The notion of pricing can become a source of controversy among health promotion professionals. One often encounters resistance to the idea of 'pricing' because it is equated with demanding money for products and/or services – typically from people least able to afford it. This is *not* what marketers have in mind when they discuss prices. Rather, pricing reflects the exchange theory basis of marketing presented earlier; that is, the mutual exchange of resources between two or more parties. Thus, prices represent the amount of resource expenditure necessary to receive desired goods or services. Prices people might consider in deciding whether to change a health behaviour or participate in a specific health promotion program include:

Geographic distance: How far is it to travel to a programme site? How convenient is it to sign up for a particular programme? How close is a safe exercise area?

Social: What will my spouse think about my quitting smoking when he still does? How will my friends react when they find out – especially the ones that smoke?

Behavioural: What am I going to do to relax if I don't smoke? What will I do when I get a craving for a cigarette?

Psychological: What if I fail to quit again? Will quitting smoking be worth the agony of withdrawal?

Physical: What if I start having strong withdrawal symptoms – what am I going to do? If I quit smoking I'll start gaining weight.

Structural: How am I going to survive at work when people are smoking everywhere in the building?

Marketers attempt to understand these and other costs from the target audience's perspective as they pose key resistance points to behaviour change. They then examine equally closely what the perceived benefits of a specific behaviour change are, and develop communication and marketing strategies that realistically address the cost issues and reinforce the benefits. Notice that cost issues are not skirted or ignored; to do so jeopardizes not only the credibility of the programme (they don't know what they're talking about!) but it is detrimental to establishing an empathy with the target group that allows them to draw the inference – 'they know what I'm going through!'

On the other side of the price equation are the 'benefits'. Again, these benefits cover the same types of categories as illustrated earlier for prices. The focus of marketers on benefits sometimes leads to segmentation strategies that are themselves based on the differing perceived benefits among the target group. For example, cigarette smokers might be segmented, not by sociodemographic factors, but by how they see the benefit of quitting: being a better role model for their children; having a healthy baby; not dying of cancer like their sibling; being able to exercise more easily; not feeling like cigarettes are controlling their life. The art of marketing lies as much in communicating effectively the benefits of behaviour change and making the 'price' worth it, as it does in production of the products to support the effort.

A focus on benefits also leads to another distinguishing characteristic of marketing programmes: their offering of incentives to motivate behaviour change. Again, there is often some resistance to the idea of 'bribing people to do something that they should do anyway' (i.e not smoke, eat right). However, many theories of behaviour change suggest that it is the anticipation of rewards – and tangible ones at that – that increases the probability of an individual engaging in the desired behaviour (Bandura 1977). Incentives have been used successfully in a number of health promotion efforts including smoking cessation campaigns (Lefebvre *et al*. 1990) and weight loss programmes (Brownell *et al*. 1984; Nelson *et al*. 1987). One need review only consumer marketing programme – the types of incentives they use and the method of promoting the desired behaviour with the incentive – to begin to recognize the many ways in which incentives can be used in a positive way to influence trials of healthy behaviours just as trials of new consumer products are promoted. A reminder to oneself that these consumer marketers spend inordinate sums of money to develop and evaluate these promotional efforts also reinforces the important formative research being engaged in by these 'competitors' that can benefit our own social marketing programmes.

Place

Place characteristics, or communication and distribution channels, have already been discussed to some extent. As with other elements of the marketing mix, decisions about 'places' need to take into account the preferences and practices of the target population. Place decisions can have an immediate impact on the accessibility of messages, products, and services to the target group. Virtually all place decisions have associated costs as well. In the discussion of 'pricing', we noted the effect place can have in terms of consumer costs (i.e. geographic price). However, at least as important are place costs borne by an organization attempting to reach specific groups. Many of these costs are fiscal (e.g. buying media time, producing flyers and brochures), but others have to do with the temporal and personnel resources necessary to achieve efficiency and effectiveness within the channel (Kotler and Andreasen 1987).

Places, or channels, are almost limitless in type. In deciding which ones to employ in a social marketing programme, the function one seeks from a channel is important. If one is choosing to communicate information, mass media may be appropriate – but should it be by television, radio, outdoor signage, transit posters, or other means? The answer lies in the results of earlier channel analysis. However, if one is interested in opening a new type of clinic service, or distributing a new health promotion product, different types of channels – for instance, retail outlets, religious organizations, kiosks – are more appropriate. Here, channel analysis may help fashion a decision, but it is likely that pilot studies will also need to be undertaken to test the feasibility and acceptability of the channel before investing many resources in the project.

The function one wishes the channel to perform in relation to a particular message/product/service and specific audience is clearly a first decision. However, other tasks that confront social marketers are then to:

Attract channel resources through direct appeals, inter-organizational agreements, co-option, financial payments, sponsorship arrangements, or development of new channels.

Co-ordinate and control the channel system, including the development of working relationships with channel gatekeepers and middlemen, ensuring that the channel system reaches the appropriate target groups, evaluating the efficacy and efficiency of the channel system and maintaining good working relationships with key gatekeepers.

Maintain the flow of messages/products/services in an orderly manner and ensure the quality of the message/product/service is maintained. This latter point can be especially critical when intermediaries are involved as happens when volunteers are deployed for certain functions, influential citizens are involved in programme awareness functions, retailers are distributing products, and media representatives are producing messages.

Promotion

Although some people equate marketing with promotion, the concept of the marketing mix puts promotional strategies in their proper context: as they relate to the product, price, and place decisions made with respect to a specific target group (Lefebvre and Floral 1988). Promotion aspects of the marketing mix involve the communication aspects of social marketing and include such strategies as advertising (either paid or public service), personal selling or contacts, public relations events, point-of purchase programmes, direct mail, telemarketing, and virtually every other opportunity the programme encounters (or can create) that puts it in front of a target group (e.g. T-shirts, balloons, newsletters, etc.). Before launching promotion after promotion however, Novelli (1984) recommends developing an overall communication strategy for a programme. Four elements need to be defined:

The *benefits* to the target group of responding to a message purchasing a product, or participating in a programme ('look better, feel great!', 'win a vacation for two!', 'feel good about yourself').

The *reasons why* the communication should be attended to and responded to by the target group ('doctors recommend . . .', 'people like you find that it works', 'more taste and less calories').

The *specific actions* the audience should undertake in response to the communication (i.e. 'call this number for more information', 'see your doctor', 'shop around the edges of supermarket').

The *tone* or *image* that should underlie all communications directed towards the public (i.e. fun and rewarding, serious and scientific, upscale and trendy).

The resulting communication strategy or concept platform (Lefebvre *et al* 1988), should concisely state these four elements. Once decisions are made about the concept platform, the 'how to' communicate questions and creative execution of each promotion can be addressed as in Table 3.

Promotion strategies can be as inexpensive or pricey as one chooses. While it is not within the capacity of many health promotion programmes, to emulate the promotional budgets of large corporate advertisers, it is sometimes the less expensive – and often more creative – efforts that have the bigger pay off in terms of actual effectiveness. Costs of promotion need to be in relation to the actual impact they have. In the commercial world, the cost of advertising is typically calculated by the reach achieved (the number of people exposed to the advertisement) – usually expressed in costs per thousand, or CPM. The reach of a promotion is calculated by such methods as independent audits of listeners or viewers (in the case of radio or television) by companies who specialize in this type of service, circulation figures adjusted for multiple readers in print media (i.e. more than one person usually reads any single copy of a newspaper or magazine on average), and random telephone surveys. Thus a mass media campaign that costs $38,180(US) and reaches 2 million people has a CPM of $0.02. However, one can raise the argument that reach, in and of itself, may not be the objective of a campaign; it may be more important to base promotion costs on actual participation rates in a programme promoted by the campaign. Thus in the example above of $38,180 spent (though donated) in mass media time, Elder *et al.* 1991) reported 802 residents enrolled in their 'Quit to Win' smoking cessation programme – for a promotion cost of $47.61 per enrollee. If one further refines the cost-effect to enrolled smokers who quit, then the media costs climb to $134.44 for each of the 284 self-reported quitters. These costs do not include 'direct' costs associated with salaries, material production, and related campaign expenses which were calculated by the authors to be $17.25 per quitter. The moral of this example is that promotional costs can be either quite inexpensive, or quite expensive, depending on the objective one sets for the effort. Clearly, a programme can reach many people rather inexpensively through the mass media, but it is not so evident that such costs are as efficient when participation rates and behaviour, change are substituted in the denominator. Unfortunately, there have been few carefully documented cost accountings of health promotion programmes to allow for meaningful and generalizable conclusions to be drawn as to which types of promotional strategies are most cost-efficient for the type of objective one sets.

Process tracking

Process tracking systems are the most important element of the implementation process once it has begun. These types of systems provide the integrative and control functions necessary for a programme manager to ensure (1) that the marketing plan is being implemented as designed, (2) that the programme is reaching its target audience, and (3) that an implementation record is maintained that can be used to modify and refine later programmes and campaigns.

In the Stanford Five City Project (Farquhar *et al.* 1990), the Minnesota Heart Health Program (Jacobs *et al.* 1986), and the Pawtucket Heart Health Program (McGraw *et al.* 1989), common needs were seen for developing tracking systems to manage and document their interventions. Each project developed a process tracking system to meet the unique needs and challenges of their intervention protocols. However, in a series of collaborative meetings, a hybrid tracking system was created that blended the major common features of each system in order to compare process tracking system data directly across the three projects (Flora *et al.* in press).

The Community Education Monitoring System (CEMS) represents a consensus of these three cardiovascular disease prevention projects as to the major elements needed in a process tracking system – again, recognizing that each project had other elements not reflected in CEMS. As such, CEMS provides a useful heuristic in designing process tracking systems for different types of programmes and settings. The major elements of CEMS are outlined in Table 8.4. They are based on a common set of assumptions and strategies shared by the three projects including:

Interventions based on a number of perspectives including social learning theory, diffusion of innovations research, social network theory, inoculation theory, social marketing, and community development models.

Multiple change objectives such as increasing public awareness and knowledge of cardiovascular risk factors, changing risk behaviours, maintaining these changes, stimulating organizational changes, and encouraging community groups to adopt particular programme elements.

The use of a variety of communication channels including electronic and print media, face-to-face and direct mail.

Multiple target audiences including high risk individuals, children, adolescents, and healthy adults.

The CEMS model is presented to stimulate research and applications in health promotion programmes of all kinds. Whether it be a CEMS-derivative, or created for other needs and necessities, process tracking systems are integral to good marketing practice. While it is difficult to imagine commercial marketers not gathering information, for instance, on how many coupons they distributed, for what specific products, and how many were redeemed (the sophisticated ones will even tell you by whom and where), it is commonplace to find health promotion organizations with only the most rudimentary and incomplete understanding of exactly what they have done and what immediate impact it had. This will have to change if we are to have well-managed and effective programmes that are sensitive to changes in the public's needs and priorities (Lefebvre and Flora 1988).

Marketing management

Implementation of a marketing orientation within an organization faces a number of potential barriers. Chief amongst these, if it is not already apparent to the reader, is that marketing programmes demand a great deal of planning and action that may be unacceptable – and actually disruptive – to the staff and organization (Lefebvre and Flora 1988). Marketing plans not only involve time, research, and turning the organization 'inside outs' to assess consumer preferences, they also require careful attention to implementation timelines, co-ordination of diverse logistics and personnel (either paid or voluntary staff), and sufficient evaluation to ascertain the plan's effectiveness in achieving preset objectives and feedforward to the

Table 8.4   Major elements of the community education monitoring system

Date of entry
Product or programme identification code
Channel
   1. Face-to-face
     a. Single session
     b. Multiple sessions
   2. Mass media
     a. Television (PSA vs. news story vs. talk show)
     b. Radio (PSA vs. programme vs. talk show)
     c. Newspaper (advertisement vs. column vs. story)
   3. Print materials
     a. Booklets
     b. Self-help kits
     c. Posters
     d. Brochures
     e. Flyers
   4. Special events
     a. Health fair
     b. Contests
     c. Training
     d. Other special activities
   5. Physical/social/political environment
     a. Smoking policies
     b. Restaurant menu-labelling
     c. Grocery store shelf-labelling
Objective of the specific intervention effort
   1. Individual change
     a. Awareness
     b. Knowledge
     c. Behaviour
   2. Organizational change
     a. Improved community relations
     b. Establishing networks
     c. Training health professionals
     d. Training lay volunteers
   3. Environmental change
     a. Policy/regulation
Target of the intervention
   1. Individuals
     a. Blood pressure
     b. Exercise
     c. Nutrition
     d. Smoking

   e. Weight control
   f. General heart health practices
2. Organizations
   a. Visibility
   b. Institutionalization

Community adoption and maintenance of interventions
   1. Percentage of activity supported by project resources
   2. Percentage of activity supported by community resources

Intervention accessibility
   1. Available to general public
   2. Available to employees/members only

Estimated reach of intervention activity
   1. Number of print pieces distributed
   2. Number of newspapers printed that day
   3. Listener/viewer share (number of households) at specific time
   4. Number of participants in activity
   5. Number of people exposed on a quarterly basis to an organizational or environmental intervention

Source: Flora *et al.* in press

next set of activities. One or more of these tasks can cause an organization to discard the marketing orientation because 'it's too hard' or 'we don't have all those resources you talk about'.

Implementing a marketing orientation, and a marketing management structure, needs to start from the top. A commitment to the process of evolving to a true market-driven agency is the first step. From there, marketing audits (see Table 8.5) can help identify current strengths and weaknesses. Focus can then be placed on addressing as many, or as few, areas as need attention with timelines for completion, and resources allocated, as the agency's other demands allow. One does not have immediately to initiate, for example, a complete database management system to begin collecting process information, nor does one have to hire professional market researchers to get input from consumers. But, as with any marketing programme described in this chapter, the 'internal' marketing plan is just as important and needs to contain achievable objectives for both the short and longterm.

Table 8.5 Outline of a marketing audit

Marketing environment

Markets
   1. Who are the organization's major markets and publics?
   2. What are the major market segments in each market?

3. What are the present and expected future size and the characteristics of each market or market segment?

Customers
1. How do the customers and public feel towards and see the organization?
2. How do customers make their purchase or adoption decisions?
3. What is the present and expected future state of consumer needs and satisfaction as they relate to the organization?

Competitors
1. Who are the organization's major competitors?
2. What trends can be foreseen in competition?

Macro-environment
1. What are the main relevant developments with respect to demography, economy, technology, government, and culture that will affect the organization's situation?

Marketing system

Objectives
1. What are the organization's long-term and short-term overall objectives and marketing objectives?
2. Are the objectives in a clear hierarchical order and in a form that permits planning and measurement of achievement?
3. Are the marketing objectives reasonable for the organization given its competitive position, resources, and opportunities?

Programme
1. What is the organization's core strategy for achieving its objectives, and is it likely to succeed?
2. Is the organization allocating enough resources (or too many) to accomplish the marketing tasks?
3. Are the marketing resources allocated optimally to the various markets, territories, and products/services of the organization?
4. Are the marketing resources allocated optimally to the major elements of the marketing mix (i.e. product development, service quality, personal contact, promotion, and distribution)?

Implementation
1. Does the organization develop an annual marketing plan? Is the planning procedure effective?
2. Does the organization implement control procedures (monthly, quarterly) to ensure that its annual plan objectives are being met?
3. Does the organization carry out periodic studies to determine the contribution and effectiveness of various marketing activities?
4. Does the organization have an adequate marketing information system (i.e. process tracking system) to service the needs of managers for planning and controlling operations in various markets?

Organization
1. Does the organization have a high-level marketing officer to analyze, plan, and implement the marketing work of the organization?
2. Are the other persons directly involved in marketing activity able people? Is there a need for more training, incentives, supervision, or evaluation?
3. Are the marketing responsibilities optimally structured to serve the needs of different marketing activities, product/service markets, and territories?

Detailed marketing activity review

Products
1. What are the main messages/products/services of the organization?
2. Should any products in the product line be phased out?
3. Should any products be added to the product line?
4. What is the general state of health of each product and the product mix as a whole?

Price
1. To what extent are prices set based on costs to the organization, consumer demand, and/or competitive criteria?
2. What would the likely response of demand be to higher or lower prices?
3. How do consumers psychologically interpret current prices?
4. Does the organization use temporary price promotions (e.g. incentives) and how effective are they?

Place
1. Are there alternative methods of distributing messages, products, and services that would result in more services or less cost?
2. Does the organization render adequate service to its customers apart from its message/product/service line?

Promotion
1. Does the organization have a communications strategy (concept platform)?
2. Does the organization allocate an appropriate amount of resources to promotional activities?
3. Are promotional themes and copy effective among the target audiences?
4. Are media well chosen? Are costs accounted for and effective for the chosen media?
5. Are direct marketing opportunities utilized to complement other promotional activities and to maintain customer contact?

Source: Adapted from Kotler 1975

The management of marketing operations within an organization involves the orchestration of organizational resources by senior management to meet consumer needs and the organization's objectives. It does not necessarily require a formal degree in marketing management to perform, yet it does require in-depth understanding of the social marketing elements and how they interrelate. It also requires good management skills and the development of an organizational culture that prizes what Dr Geoffrey Rose has been quoted as describing as 'Dirty hands and clean minds'. That is, the ability of staff to work in the field, staying directly in touch with their clients and getting things done while also being able to exercise the critical and strategic cognitive skills that make a good scientist. There may be no better definition of a social marketer.

Fashioning an organization that is market-orientated may require an elaboration of existing staff roles and functions. In the work of the Pawtucket Heart Health Program's Intervention Unit, eight key functions were identified, and organizational structure and staff responsibilities were modified accordingly. These functions included:

Product development, within which specific staff had responsibility for development, testing, implementation, evaluation, and refinement of intervention messages, products, and services within their areas of risk behaviour change expertise (i.e. smoking cessation, blood pressure control, weight loss, blood cholesterol management, and physical activity). These staff assumed titles of 'product manager' for each intervention programme, and, as in the corporate sector, these product managers were delegated ultimate authority and responsibility for their product line, including the development of annual marketing plans for each product.

Training, in which specific staff with training expertise were designated as trainers for both paid and unpaid staff in various skills, including blood pressure measurement, blood cholesterol measurement, and dietary counselling, and group leaders for smoking cessation and weight loss programmes. These trainers were also responsible for supervision of volunteer staff in each of these areas, monitored service quality, and did annual recertification examinations of knowledge and skills for each staff person active in these programmes.

Channel development responsibilities for other staff not designated as product managers. Channels identified by the Intervention Unit for which one staff person had responsibility included worksites, religious organizations, mass media, and those channels through which the minority populations of Pawtucket could be reached most effectively (targeted radio and print media, religious organizations in those neighbourhoods, worksites with high ratios of minority employees, food retail outlets, and specific housing developments). These 'channel managers' developed and nurtured relationships with gatekeepers in their channel area, and worked with product managers in establishing distribution of messages, products, and services to meet organizational objectives of the project.

Resource development was most prominent in the project through recruitment of lay volunteers in the community. Again, specific staff – designated as the 'Volunteer Team' – made many contacts with community groups through which to recruit volunteers. They worked with product managers to identify staffing needs (e.g. weight loss group leaders), developed marketing plans to recruit and maintain volunteer staff, and managed the volunteer registry that enabled them to match emerging programme needs with expertise and talents of volunteers already involved in the project (see Roncarati *et al*. 1989 for more details about this process). Resource development also included assignment of staff to locate financial resources as well from local businesses, as when incentives were needed for major behaviour change campaigns or new product development.

Promotion for all products had in-house resource staff assigned to it including editorial and graphic services supported by desk-top publishing expertise in the Administrative Unit. All work went through this group to ensure that the project's concept platform and image were reinforced through the packaging and tone of the materials.

Programme delivery as a key function was defined by product managers who worked with their own volunteer staff to reach city residents with behaviour change programmes. Participant registries were managed by staff and telephone and mail follow-up to people identified at risk for cardiovascular disease through screening, counselling, and referral programmes was an important element of the programme delivery process.

Management of the marketing programme was overseen by the Unit Co-ordinator, but occurred at a variety of levels in the organization. All staff had areas of management responsibility, whether it was products, channels, and/or resources. Annual two-day planning retreats and a mid-year one-day staff retreat to evaluate progress across the specific product marketing plans were important elements in co-ordinating staff efforts through the setting of annual objectives for the entire Unit which then drove the product planning process.

Evaluation of the intervention process was carried out through staff in the Formative and Process Evaluation section of the project's Evaluation Unit. The evaluation staff worked with product managers in testing new products and their efficacy in reaching target populations and promoting behaviour change amongst participants. This group also managed the programme's process evaluation system that monitored the Intervention Unit activities and is reflected in the earlier discussion of the CEMS. Readers interested in more details about the formative and process evaluation system may refer to McGraw *et al*. 1989.

These eight functions do not necessarily have to be translated into at least eight full-time staff positions in order for an organization to become effective in marketing. Rather, the organization should review its current staffing pattern and areas of responsibility with these points in mind. One staff person may have responsibilities that cut across several functions, and, indeed, in the Pawtucket Heart Health Program we approached each staff position as a mixture of each of these functions, with varying weights assigned to each one; for instance, volunteer team members were responsible for managing volunteer-related products and services, including marketing plans, were involved in promotion activities, and managed their own groups of volunteers. However, it is important that each of the areas receives an allotment of staff time for a fully functioning marketing operation.

Managing to market, versus managing for managing's sake, may also bring health promotion organizations to the point of evolving new management practices that reflect a very different world from the one we have been used to in the past. This new world, characterized by such trends as rapid and accelerating change, more consumer control over how they allocate their time, component lifestyles, an ageing population in developed countries, increasing globalization of many human endeavours, and changing work environments, requires new management strategies for organizations to survive, and even thrive, in it (Lefebvre in press). Proposed management evolutions to meet these new demands and challenges note that dynamism, not control, is necessary for effective action and response. Flattened hierarchies, not more management layers, will ensure organizational responsiveness and closer touch with consumers. Fluidity in team building and development, as opposed to highly organized and sharply demarcated areas of responsibility, will encourage innovative approaches by staff to the new challenges of health promotion. Pushing responsibility and authority down in the organization, not centralizing them, will empower staff to make things happen and focus on consumers as the critical link – not what the boss thinks! Leadership by example, rather than by fiat, will further inspire greater efforts by staff. And finally, measuring what is important for success, not just what is convenient and measurable, will allow health promotion professionals to set their sites on the real objectives and goals necessary to fashion a healthier population (Lefebvre in press; Peters 1987).

CONCLUDING REMARKS

Social marketing is garnering much attention from public health professionals with an accompanying enthusiasm that it offers a new 'magic bullet' with which we can address social and health problems. While there are many success stories as to how social marketing principles led to significant and impressive results, it must also be recognized that these case studies lack the rigour of empirical investigations. Thus, while promising, one cannot – nor should not – suggest that social marketing is the health promoter's panacea. Many questions still remain.

There are numerous research questions that need to be addressed in social marketing. What is most unfortunate about this state of affairs is that it has changed very little in the ten years since Bloom and Novelli (1981) surveyed the area. Some of the issues and questions they raised then have received scant attention since; amongst the more salient are:

The difficulty in funding and completing consumer research studies in a timely fashion.

The lack of behavioural data on which to base segmentation strategy, and the related challenge that few data are available as to which segmentation strategies are most appropriate for specific target behaviours.

The formulation of messages, products, and services is hampered by the intangible quality of much of what health promotion is attempting to market and the scientific, social, and political context of many problems that require compromise, and at worst inaction, on important health concerns.

In the area of pricing, the pressure is on social marketers only to reduce costs, due in part to the lack of information and models about how consumers view costs and benefits associated with health promotive behaviours.

The difficulties associated with using intermediaries for much of our work, again due to a lack of understanding as to how to employ incentives appropriately to ensure co-operation and maintenance of quality.

Communication strategies that are often driven by needs to communicate relatively large amounts of information but are restricted on such complete disclosures because of the nature of preferred media (i.e. television), the inaccessibility of paid advertising due to resource limitations, and pressures not to use certain types of appeals or 'tell the whole story'.

It is bringing together the practitioners of the art of social marketing with the scientists who can test and evaluate the approach that is the critical need at this time. Such a partnership requires that agencies who fund research look towards a more balanced portfolio in which the more 'pure' investigational studies (such as are found in much basic and clinical research) are complemented by the more 'dirty' work of understanding in the real world context how to translate new scientific knowledge into messages, products, and services that will improve the health and well-being of people everywhere. Social marketing may provide the type of strategic and practical tools with which Health For All can be achieved; it is incumbent on each of us to assure that it is applied appropriately and wisely.

REFERENCES

Bandura, A. (1977) *Social Learning Theory*, Englewood Cliffs, NJ: Prentice–Hall.

Bloom, P. N. and Novelli, W. D. (1981) 'Problems and challenges of social marketing', *Journal of Marketing* 45: 79–88.

Brownell, K. D., Cohen, R. Y., Stunkard, A. J., Felix, M. R. J., and Cooley, N. (1984) 'Weight loss competitions at the worksite: impact on weight, morale, and cost-effectiveness', *American Journal of Public Health* 74: 1283–5.

Doremus Porter Novelli (1986) *Lessons Learned from the DuaLima Test Market*, Washington, DC: SOMARC/The Futures Group.

Elder, J. P., Campbell, N. R., Mielchen, S. D., Hovell, M. F., and Litrownik, A. J. (1991) 'Implementation and evaluation of a community-sponsored smoking cessation contest', *American Journal of Health Promotion* 5: 200–7.

Farquhar, J. W., Fortmann, S. P., Flora, J. A., Taylor, C. B., Haskell, W. L., Williams, P. T., Maccoby, N., and Wiid, P. D. (1990) 'Effects of communitywide education on cardiovascular disease risk factors: the Stanford Five-City Project', *Journal of the American Medical Association* 264: 359–65.

Fine, S. H. (1981) *The Marketing of Ideas and Social Issues*, New York: Praeger.

Flora, J. A., Lefebvre, R. C., Murray, D. M., Stone, E. J., Assaf, A., Mittelmark, M., and Finnegan, J. R. (in press) 'A community education monitoring system: methods from the Stanford Five-City Project, the Minnesota Heart Health Program, and the Pawtucket Heart Health Program', *Health Education Research: Theory and Practice*.

Jacobs, Jr., D. R., Luepker, R. V., Mittelmark, M. B., Folson, A. R., Pirie, P. L., Mascioli, S. R., Hannan, P. J., Pechacek, T. F., Bracht, N. F., Carlaw, R. W., Kline, F. G., and Blackburn, H. (1986) 'Community-wide prevention strategies: evaluation design of the Minnesota Heart Health Program', *Journal of Chronic Disease* 39: 775–88.

Kotler, P. (1975) *Marketing for Nonprofit Organizations*, Englewood Cliffs, NJ: Prentice-Hall.

Kotler, P. and Andreasen, A. R. (1987) *Strategic Marketing for Nonprofit Organizations*, 3rd edition, Englewood Cliffs, NJ: Prentice-Hall.

Kotler, P. and Bloom, P. N. (1984) *Marketing Professional Services*, Englewood Cliffs, NJ: Prentice-Hall.

Kotler, P. and Roberto, E. L. (1989) *Social Marketing: Strategies for Changing Public Behavior*, New York: The Free Press.

Kotler, P. and Zaltman, G. (1971) 'Social marketing: an approach to planned social change', *Journal of Marketing* 35: 3–12.

Lefebvre, R. C. (1990) 'Strategies to maintain and institutionalize successful programs: a marketing framework', in N. Bracht (ed.) *Health Promotion at the Community Level*, Newburg Park, CA: Sage.

—— (in press) 'Consumer trends in the 1990s: implications for health promotion', *American Journal of Health Promotion*.

Lefebvre, R. C. and Flora, J. A. (1988) 'Social marketing and public health intervention', *Health Education Quarterly* 15: 299–315.

Lefebvre, R. C., Lasater, T. M., Carleton, R. C., and Peterson, G. (1986) 'Theory and practice of health programming in the community: the Pawtucket Heart Health Program', *Preventive Medicine* 16: 80–95.

Lefebvre, R. C., Harden, E. A., and Zompa, B. (1988) 'The Pawtucket Heart Health Program: III. social marketing to promote community health', *Rhode Island Medical Journal* 71: 27–30.

Lefebvre, R. C., Cobb, G. D., Goreczny, A. J., and Carleton, R. A. (1990)

'Efficacy of an incentive-based community smoking cessation program', *Addictive Behaviors* 15: 403–11.

McGraw, S. A., McKinlay, S. M., McClements, L., Lasater, T. M., Assaf, A., and Carleton, R. A. (1989) 'Methods in program evaluation: the process evaluation system of the Pawtucket Heart Health Program', *Evaluation Review* 13: 459–83.

McGuire, W. J. (1984) 'Public communication: a strategy for inducing health promoting behavior change', *Preventive Medicine* 18: 299–319.

Manoff, R. K. (1985) *Social Marketing*, New York: Praeger.

Nelson, D. J., Sennett, L., Lefebvre, R. C., Loiselle, L., McClements, L., and Carleton, R. A. (1987) 'A campaign strategy for weight loss at worksites', *Health Education Research: Theory and Practice* 2: 27–31.

Novelli, W. D. (1984) 'Developing marketing programs', in L. W. Frederickson, L. J. Solomon, and K. A. Brehony (eds) *Marketing Health Behavior: Principles, Techniques and Applications*, New York: Plenum.

Peters, T. (1987) *Thriving on Chaos: Handbook for a Management Revolution*, New York: Knopf.

Rice, R. E. and Atkin, C. K. (1989) 'Trends in communication campaign research', in R. E. Rice and C. K. Atkin (eds) *Public Communication Campaigns*, 2nd edition, Newbury Park, CA: Sage.

Rogers, E. M. (1983) *Diffusion of Innovations*, New York: The Free Press.

Roncarati, D. D., Lefebvre, R. C., and Carleton, R. A. (1989) 'Voluntary involvement in community health promotion: the Pawtucket Heart Health Program', *Health Promotion* 4: 11–18.

Weinstein, A. (1987) *Market Segmentation*, Chicago, IL: Probus.

Chapter 9

Communication theory and health promotion

Gordon Macdonald

Communication at its very simplest involves a communicator or communication event, a message, and a recipient. This communication act is the basic building block for all social relationships. It is the means by which all information and knowledge is transmitted. The communicator uses a series of signs or symbols which he or she encodes in a message. The recipient, once his or her attention is aroused, decodes the message and, if motivated, acts on the information received. In essence the communication event is to do with the conveyance of meaning. The effectiveness of any given message influences the degree to which it is decoded and acted upon. Communication used in this sense is as much to do with persuasion as it is to do with informing: it is not therefore to be confused with communication in an educational sense (see Chapter 4). It is more akin to training (as in education and training) since it attempts to develop certain attitudes and forms of behaviour. A great deal of research has gone into the development of persuasive communication and a useful bibliography lists over 25,000 studies (Lipstein and McGuire 1978).

The simplistic model of communication noted above is developed into something much more substantial by McGuire (1978). In his persuasion/communication matrix he cites five communication or input variables (see Figure 9.1) which further develop the three outlined above. Each of these five input variables, source, message, channel, receiver, and destination, can be subdivided again into four, five, or even six further dependent variables. The variables contributing to source, for example, could be credibility, likeability, power, quantity, and demography; or to message they could be appeal, style, organization, and quantity; to channel they would be mass media, directness (essentially one-to-one), and human sensory modes; to receiver they would be demographic characteristics, personality traits, and receiver attitude/belief characteristics; and finally to destination (in the sense of the ultimate goal of the communication) they would be cognitive/behavioural targets and whether the final impact was product or practice based.

On the vertical axis of the matrix six output variables are listed which are a great deal less controllable than the input variables. These independent

Input: Communication variables	Source				Message					Channel	Receiver	Destination
Output: Steps in being persuaded	Credibility	Likability	Power	Quantity	Demographics	Appeal	Style	Organization	Quantity			
Exposure												
Simple exposure												
Attention to communication												
Emotional Response												
Arousal												
Affect												
Encoding												
Attention to content												
Perception												
Learning												
Remembering												
Acceptance												
Overt Behaviour												
Consolidation												

(See text for details of columns and rows subdivisions)

Figure 9.1 The communication/persuasion matrix, indicating the divisions on the input (communication) side and on the output (persuasion) side

Source: Lipstein and McGuire 1978

variables include exposure to the message (if the communication is to have any persuasive impact at all); second, information perception; third, the essentials of the communication must be decoded (comprehended and stored); fourth, the message must be acceptable; fifth, overt behaviour in line with the communicator's intent must follow; and finally there should be some form of post-behavioural consolidation. The matrix may be viewed in terms of the vertical axis representing the persuasion output and the horizontal axis representing the communication input. In very general terms and accepting a non-linear progression the further down and to the right the communication goes the more successful it becomes. In other words when the communication has reached the consolidation/destination intersection then it has reached the intended extent of the message originator. McGuire's persuasion/communication matrix represents a scheme for understanding the psychological, physical, and spatial considerations associated with communication even though it may be criticized for breaking up what is a continuous and on-going process into fragmented boxed sections. This process is of crucial importance if the communication is concerned with a new idea, practice, or product since it is the intention of the communicator to promote adoption of the innovation. Effective communication and the diffusion and adoption of new ideas and practices should be essential features in all health promotion programmes. Innovation-diffusion theory as a distinct branch of wider communication theories can offer a valuable contribution to the theoretical base for health education and health promotion. This chapter will describe the critical features of innovation-diffusion theory, propose some criticism of it, and yet show, with the aid of one or two examples, how it can be of use in the broader development of health promotion as a discipline.

INNOVATION-DIFFUSION THEORY

The origins of innovation-diffusion research and discipline development can be traced back to the nineteenth century when British and German social anthropologists developed forms of diffusion theory in attempting to explain why a particular society adopts new practices and ideas. These theories were picked up by the French sociologist Tarde (1903) who pioneered the 'S'-shaped diffusion curve and the idea of the pivotal role of opinion leaders. However, it was not until the middle of the twentieth century that a truly new paradigm emerged with the publication of a study on the diffusion of a new hybrid corn in Iowa by Ryan and Gross (1943). This study is referred to again later in this chapter, but it is worth noting at this stage that, although diffusion research is a particular type or branch of communication research, it mostly developed in academic departments, such as psychology, anthropology, and sociology. Until the 1960s there were few, if any, departments specializing in communication studies anywhere in the world. The classical 'model' developed for the communication of innovations identifies four key elements, namely an innovation (1) which is communicated through certain channels (2) over a period of time (3) to members of a social system (4) (Schramm and Lerner 1978).

An innovation has been defined (Rogers 1983) as an idea or practice or object perceived as new by an individual. It is the perceived newness of the idea that largely determines the individual's reaction to it. It matters little to the individual just how objectively new an idea or practice is. Robertson (1971) however attempted to define degrees of newness or innovation. A continuous innovation causes the least disruption of the conventional consumption patterns of a community or individual. Examples of a continuous innovation, in the context of health promotion, are adding fluoride to toothpaste or reducing sugar content in jam. A dynamically continuous innovation involves more disruption than a continuous innovation; it need not involve new consumption patterns but it often involves a new product that alters behaviour in some way, for example an electric tooth-brush. Finally, a discontinuous innovation is one that involves a new product or practice and involves new consumption patterns and forms of behaviour. Examples here might be exercise bicycles, television, or aerobics.

This categorization of Robertson's is more applicable to commercial products rather than to innovation in terms of behaviour related to health. Even the distinction by Brown (1981) between a consumer innovation like a television set and a technological innovation like robotic production lines does little to clarify the situation. In relation to this chapter the author is far more interested in an innovation that concerns new forms of behaviour and practices, particularly in how they apply to health, as opposed to product innovation, although the latter may well accompany new forms of lifestyle. Innovation-diffusion theory and practice can then be related back to basic communication theory.

Innovation requires communication. In the basic model of source — message — recipient, outlined at the beginning of the chapter, the message element as well as the recipient becomes of paramount importance. With an innovation there is introduced a degree of uncertainty since to the individual recipient the message is the innovation and therefore subjectively new. This is the unique and peculiar nature of diffusion of innovations.

Diffusion on the other hand is the process by which an innovation is communicated. The diffusion is communicated by a variety of channels over a period of time within a social system or community. It is a process of convergence rather than divergence, that is, it is concerned with a two-way flow of communication between the source of the innovation and the recipient of it. Diffusion is, as a result, concerned with social change, since when new ideas are forthcoming and disseminated they are either adopted or rejected, both of which lead to certain consequences, and social change is likely to occur.

The classical model of diffusion (briefly referred to above) identified four main elements or constituents of diffusion. These four elements are

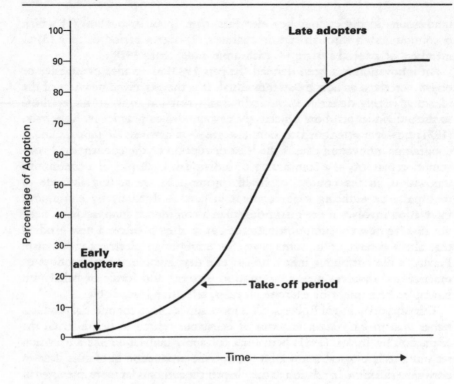

Figure 9.2   The S-shaped diffusion curve

common to all diffusion research. They are (1) the innovation, (2) the communication channels, (3) the time lapse, and (4) the social system or community (Figure 9.2).

Similarly any communication of innovations is subject to generalization relating to the nature of the communication and the speed with which it is adopted, evaluated, and accepted. Rogers and Shoemaker (1971) have derived a set of 103 generalizations from major research projects on adoption-diffusion and produced an adoption model based on four functional stages. These stages summarized below relate to traditional approaches or models in diffusion studies.

Rogers and Shoemaker	*Traditional*
1. Knowledge	1. Awareness
	2. Information
2. Persuasion	3. Evaluation
3. Decision	4. Trial adoption
4. Adoption (or rejection)	5. Adoption

The traditional model first conceptualized by rural sociologists at Iowa State University (Ryan and Gross 1943) consists of five stages. The awareness stage for the individual is characterized by the fact that s/he first learns of the innovation, but has no detailed knowledge. At the second stage the person seeks further information about the innovation and possibly considers usage. The evaluation stage could mean the mental adoption by the individual. This would involve weighing up the pros and contra-indications for adoption. The next stage includes the trial of the innovation (in some small way) to determine its value. At the final adoption stage the individual would decide whether to use the innovation on a large scale or not.

Rogers and Shoemaker's model makes one or two modifications. First, their knowledge stage is essentially a combining of the awareness and information process from the traditional model. The persuasion stage is characterized by the individual attempting to form favourable or unfavourable attitudes towards the innovation. The recipient then engages in activities designed to test the acceptability of the idea (decision stage) and this loosely relates to the trial adoption stage, but it is at the fourth stage that Rogers and Shoemaker's model deviates the most radically from the traditional approaches in that they build into it the distinct possibility of rejection or discontinuity and this is a useful contribution.

Both models rely heavily on the rational conceptualization of decision making (knowledge leads to attitude shift leads to changed practice or adoption) and not necessarily on human motivation or behaviour in the real world. The stages are not necessarily sequential either, in that the individual may evaluate without first seeking knowledge or may trial adopt before going through the persuasion/evaluation stage. Similarly an individual may lose interest and reject the innovation at any stage rather that wait until the final stage as indicated in both models. Perhaps a more realistic model is illustrated in Figure 9.3. Whilst it represents a sequential course for the individual during the diffusion there is more flexibility in it and it does allow movement between any of the stages or indeed stage omissions.

Whichever model is adopted and whichever sequence is followed by the individual the whole adoption process is something of a mental exercise for anyone exposed to an innovation; that is, the individual passes through a series of stages relating to adoption-diffusion from when first learning of the new idea to its final adoption.

There are however three other important mitigating factors associated with adoption-diffusion: time, information source, and acceptance variables.

For many innovations an S-shaped curve has characterized full diffusion. Ryan and Gross demonstrated in their study of the adoption of hybrid seed corn within a farming community that it took fourteen years for the product to be fully accepted and adopted and that the cumulative adoption percentage followed the S-shape with a five-year lag period between awareness and adoption (Figure 9.4).

The information source is a second contributory factor in determining not only the rate of adoption but also the speed of communication and credibility

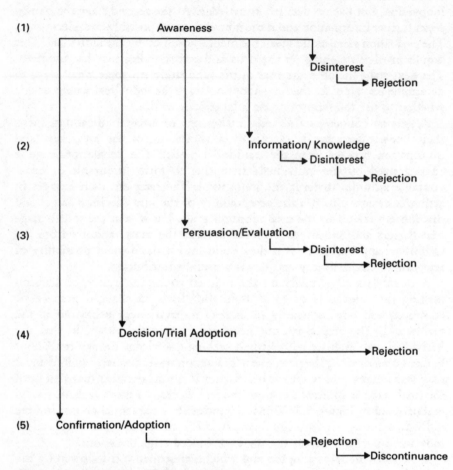

Figure 9.3 Innovation-diffusion stages

attached to the innovation. Specific information sources relate more closely to particular stages of adoption. Mass media, crucially television, play an important role in the early stages concerned with information and awareness but are less significant in the later stages. Here interpersonal sources such as friends and known experts become far more important and are considered critical during the evaluation and the (trial) adoption stages. This construct was supported by Yarbrough *et al.* (1970) when they too examined rank orders of information sources reported by farmers in the Midwest of the USA. It also lends weight to the argument that mass media serve to inform and raise awareness admirably but they have limited effect in changing opinions or behaviour.

Acceptance variables that might influence the degree or rate at which an innovation is taken up are numerous but may be divided roughly into

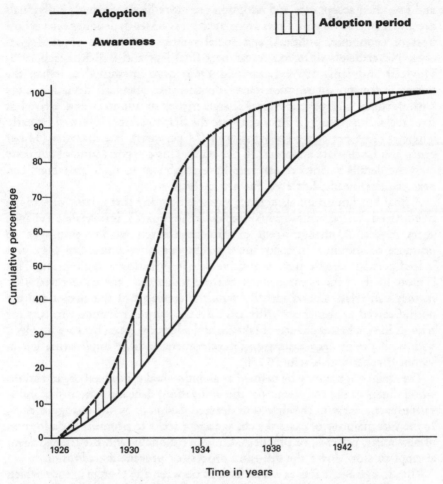

Figure 9.4 Adoption of hybrid seed corn in two Iowa farm communities
Source: Ryan and Gross 1943

social structure variables and individual characteristics. Social structures or systems can play a critical role in determining the speed of diffusion. If the system norm and the hierarchical structure are such that innovation is encouraged then acceptance rates will be higher than in a more traditional static structure. Similarly, if the directive for change is imposed from the top rather than allowing a 'free market' approach to the innovation or an approach that involves consensus and elaborate conferring, then the change will be most rapid.

Individual character variables vary the rate of acceptance principally in two ways. First, if the individual perceives the innovation as having a clearly recognizable advantage over existing practices in terms of cognition and use, then acceptance and adoption are more likely. Second, individuals accept change at varying times from awareness onset depending on a whole host of economic, political, and social reasons as well as psychological ones. Nevertheless diffusion researchers (DeFleur and Ball-Rokeach 1975; Hovland and Janis 1959; Lazarsfeld 1963) have attempted to relate the normal diffusion distribution curve divided into standard deviation units with personal and psychological characteristics of adopters and arrived at five labels. Innovators (2.5 per cent) are the first to adopt, followed by early adopters (13.5 per cent), early majority (34 per cent), late majority (34 per cent), and finally late adopters (16 per cent). This categorization of adopters (and the details various researchers have attributed to their characters and personalities) needs, however, further analysis.

A final but important acceptance variable and one that relates very much to health education/promotion diffusion is the apparent importance a change agent makes. A change agent or project/research worker employed to promote or monitor an innovation practice or programme can play, and indeed perhaps should play, a positive role in diffusion and adoption. This is more likely if the agent is client-centred rather than agency-centred: that is, they can relate to and identify with the concerns of the clients and are not perceived as somehow 'different'. This is why curriculum projects for schools have a better chance of take up and adoption if teachers are involved with both the project writing and development and the implementation in school (Becher and Maclure 1978).

The change agent may be defined as an individual (or indeed organization) who influences the recipients' (of the innovation) decisions about that innovation particularly in the direction deemed desirable by the change agency. In the vast majority of cases the change agent seeks to promote the adoption of new ideas, policies, or practices. Only occasionally will the change agent attempt to slow down the diffusion process or prevent the adoption.

The change agent acts as a kind of link between the change agency which developed the innovation (or promoted its dissemination) and the recipient of the innovation, often referred to as the client, or client system since it may be an organization and not an individual. However, if there was no social or technical difference between the change agency and the client system, then there would be little need for a change agent. One of the principal tasks of the change agent is to mediate and reduce the differences that exist between the agency and the client. These differences centre around the degrees of technical expertise available within the change agency compared to that available in the client system, what Rogers (1983) has referred to as heterophily. In many cases it can cause problems for the change agent since their loyalties may be divided between the change agency and the client. Nevertheless, if the innovation is to be successfully diffused, then the change agent is a key link. The agent must however display and exhibit certain characteristics if the diffusion process is to succeed. First, the change agent should attempt to reduce the degree of heterophily between agency and client by developing homophily with the client system or individuals within that system. This may mean in practice that the agent positively seeks out those individuals who are similar in class, status, and educational attainment to themselves (Roling *et al.* 1976). Second, whilst the change agent may need to empathize with clients and the client agency, the degree of success in the diffusion process is much more likely to depend on the rate of effort the agent puts into the communication activities (Fliegel 1966). Third, change agents need to make continued contact with all types of adoption categories within the client system if the diffusion process is to be comprehensive. In an agricultural diffusion study in Brazil (Rogers *et al.* 1970) contact with potential adopters was made up as follows:

Innovators	20
Early adopters	15
Early majority	12
Late majority	5
Laggards	3

Change agent contact is an important variable in innovation-diffusion. This contact does however tend to go through seven key stages no matter what the nature of the diffusion or the type of client system. The first stage is to do with developing awareness of needs in the client; there must be a need for change. The second stage is, or can be, time consuming in that it involves building client trust in the agent. This is an essential precursor to acceptance of an innovation. Third, the change agent should convert the expressed needs of the client into some form of diagnosis to facilitate the innovation-diffusion process. The fourth stage involves promoting the intent to change, a kind of behavioural intention in the client, with the fifth stage converting that intention into action. Having introduced the adoption, the sixth stage involves ensuring its survival within the client system and prevent discontinuance. Finally, the seventh and last stage is the ending of the working relationship between change agent and client. This is difficult but should involve allowing the client to become self-reliant and, in a sense, their own change agent.

Change agents are, then, critical components of the innovation-diffusion process. But decisions centred around whether to adopt an innovation or not are also determined by the social system or context within which the decision has to be made. Those decisions can either be individual ones or may be made by some form of authority on behalf of individuals or groups within the system or indeed by groups themselves in the form of a collective decision. Diffusion will probably be most rapid if the decision is authority imposed (Havelock 1974). This is because the decision to accept or reject an innovation is made by a relatively few powerful individuals in a system (organization) who have some 'right' to impose the innovation. The rate of adoption is likely to be slowest with a collective decision because of the need for consensus and close co-ordinated behaviour within the group. Individual or optional decision making concerning an innovation would come somewhere in between and would be affected by such influences as social norms, peer pressure, or communication networks.

Some innovation decision-making processes are in fact a combination of all three types outlined above. For example, the introduction of seat belts in the UK was based on optional decision making: manufacturers and individual car users could decide individually whether to adopt them or not. Legislation was then introduced making car manufacturers include seat belts in cars, although most car manufacturers had already made a collective decision to do this. Finally in 1983 an authority-based decision was taken making the wearing of seat belts by car drivers compulsory.

HEALTH PROMOTION PROJECTS AND INNOVATION-DIFFUSION

Innovation-diffusion is, then, an integral and important component of a more general body of communication theory and can play a unique bridging role in developing the health promoter's understanding of communication theory and techniques. If we consider the introduction of new health promotion curriculum material into schools we can see the application of diffusion theory to health-promotion practice. The inventor(s) or writer(s) of the material may be considered the innovator and the material itself the innovation. The method by which this is promoted to teachers or schools would act as the communication channel; the time period might be one day, one term, or even an academic year, and the social system would be the school or perhaps a local education authority (LEA) or indeed a consortium of LEAs. Each school or LEA would go through the functional stages outlined above and decide whether to adopt or discontinue with the material (the innovation) and this would largely depend on support from the opinion leaders (headteachers, advisory teachers, or health promotion co-ordinators) and from the change agents (local or national health promotion agencies or advisory teachers). Ultimately, schools will exhibit the uptake characteristics outlined by Rogers (1983) and fall into one of five categories: innovators, early adopters, early majority, late majority, and laggards.

This outline was followed with the development of many school-based health promotion curriculum projects, including the Schools Council Health Education Project materials, the Free to Choose teaching pack, and more recently the Skills for Adolescence and the Drugwise packs both produced by the Teachers' Advisory Council for Alcohol and Drug Misuse (TACADE). A recent survey indicated that where good dissemination methods had prevailed then the likelihood of continuance with the materials was high (Parcel et al. 1989). In this study the researchers studied the diffusion and uptake of the Minnesota Smoking Prevention Programme (MSPP) in the States and found that the innovatory programme was more likely to be adopted because it was easy to understand, it appeared superior to existing smoking prevention programmes, and it generated visible results even on a trial basis. Similar claims have been made in the UK with the Family Smoking Education project (FSE) (Newman and Nutbeam 1989; Ledwith and Peers 1988). Two studies measuring school awareness of the innovation (FSE) and factors influencing the adoption of the material (Project Smoke Free Education Group) show that the adoption rate is likely to be affected by the homophily of the change agency. That is, where the material was distributed and disseminated by a local change agent the likelihood of adoption and maintenance was high.

The Working with Groups (WWG) package, developed in the early 1980s in the UK, experienced a classical S-shaped diffusion curve during its dissemination (final report TACADE 1986). The WWG was innovatory because it provided a tangible product and skill for health education and health promotion specialists at a time when there was only a limited appreciation of the need to specialize. The innovators, the authors of the training package, ran a two-day workshop designed to familiarize the attendees with the material. At this stage the potential early adopters could show lack of interest and reject the innovation, but, after evaluation and revision, the package was enthusiastically received by the original attendees. Diffusion of the materials then commenced in earnest. Regional co-ordinators for the dissemination of the package were appointed and trained; they then became, in a sense, the change agents. They were regionally (or locally) based and so exhibited a degree of homophily with potential users of the materials. Dissemination of the training package took place over the next two years with some startling results. All regions in the UK were exposed to the material and by the end of 1986 over 700 people had taken part in the training workshops and gone on, in turn, to run similar dissemination courses. The WWG package was adopted on a large scale by health education and promotion specialists and became one of the most popular resource materials used by this professional group. There were a few reasons why this was achieved. First, the package was easily understood and usable; second, it could be adapted to circumstance, that is, used in its entirety, in part, or in conjunction with other material; third, the role of the regional co-ordinators was vital in the cascade approach to the innovation-diffusion through the classical train-the-trainers methodology; fourth, the participatory nature of the materials made it more comprehensible (Macdonald 1986); and, fifth, the network of regional co-ordinators allowed for the sharing of experience and expertise which provided support and development.

Innovation-diffusion theory does have, then, important implications for the dissemination of health promotion projects at local and national levels but it also provides a valuable contribution to health promotion as a discipline (Portnoy et al. 1989). There are, however, important caveats and it might be worth considering some of the problems associated with diffusion theory and research before concluding the chapter.

LIMITATIONS TO DIFFUSION THEORY

Communication of innovation theory relies heavily on research studies around product diffusion, whether applied to the commercial world or within the ambit of public health policy and health promotion. Research into the dissemination and diffusion of particular health promotion materials within a community intervention programme is fraught with methodological difficulties relating to *research design, measurement, and analysis*. This chapter is not concerned with the relative merits of using cross-sectional, quasi-experimental, or case study research designs since the merits of each are dealt with extensively elsewhere (Nutbeam *et al.* 1990; Puska *et al.* 1985; Maccoby *et al.* 1977 and indeed to some extent in this book (see Chapter 5) but there are cautionary tales associated with research design. Essentially, because health promotion projects and programmes are, by their very nature, dynamic and because there are still large knowledge gaps in the study of diffusion within health promotion programmes, it is better to use *prospective studies*, or at least a *combination of research designs*, when developing research methodology.

In relation to *measurement*, diffusion research is criterion referenced rather than norm referenced in general. That is, when researchers measure diffusion they tend to use pre-established criteria and not comparative data between social systems. For example, a health promotion intervention that was designed to promote weight loss within a community setting is normally measured in terms of how it compares to a pre-determined standard rather than how it compares to a similar intervention in a workplace setting.

Second, in relation to *analysis*, the focus tends to be on individual outcome factors (Green and Lewis 1986) rather than on larger organizational or social issues such as network analysis. Here as much attention is paid to tracing the progress of the communication of an innovation, investigating such issues as interpretation of the innovation, distortion of the communication, etc., as there is to the eventual quantitative outcome (Hannon and Zucker 1989).

There are however other criticisms of innovation-diffusion theory and research, and one of the most serious is the *pro-innovation bias* of researchers (Schramm and Lerner 1978). Here there is an assumption by theorists and researchers that the innovation is a 'good' thing, and should be adopted by everyone. Research methodology has been built around the assumption that innovation is good and so in a way method has followed a non-null hypothesis. Research on innovation-diffusion is often concerned with descriptive analysis of what is rather than what could be. In other words there has been little attempt at testing alternative practices through some kind of quasi-case control study. Pro-innovation researchers also fail to take into account issues to do with lack of awareness or ignorance of the innovation, to play down discontinuance of an innovation (see Figure 9.2), or they fail to look at anti-diffusion programmes which are designed to prevent or slow down socially unacceptable new practices (e.g. drug taking). There are two principal reasons for this: first that much diffusion research, in both the USA and the UK at least, is funded by those agencies, essentially change agencies, that have an interest in promoting innovation: second, those innovations that are highly visible or 'successful' provide a rate of adoption that the researchers can analyse. Obviously an innovation that hasn't been adopted leaves little for researchers to investigate.

Coupled with this pro-innovation bias in diffusion studies is the issue of individual blame bias or victim blaming (similar to the approach used in many early health education programmes). So pro-innovation research bias is reinforced with victim-blaming approaches to assess the adoption of innovations because it is assumed that the innovation is 'good' and should be adopted. Those that do not adopt are labelled 'inadequate' through the use of a number of variables, such as income, educational standards, social class, cosmopolitanism or exposure to mass media. This emphasis on the individual at the expense of the system has clouded many of the diffusion studies undertaken principally in the United States (Rogers 1983). System blame (the system is responsible to some extent for the decisions behind adoption or rejection of innovations by individuals) might allow for greater objectivity in diffusion research. Caplan and Nelson (1973) argue that diffusion researchers get confused between cause of an event or condition, which should be subject to scientific evaluation, and blame for an event or condition, which is subject to values and opinions. Often these values and opinions are those of the researcher or investigator. Blame is more easily attributable to an individual and as most communication research is conducted at the individual unit level, with the possible exception of anthropological studies, it is not surprising that diffusion research adopts a victim-blaming approach in cases where innovation is rejected or ignored.

One of the principal problems associated with the communication of innovation is *time*. In studying a process like diffusion time is a key ingredient but also a methodological nightmare. Diffusion of innovations takes time and as such either requires well-constructed longitudinal research which pays close attention to process elements within the diffusion or relies heavily on participant recall. Unfortunately most diffusion studies rely on the latter method (Basch *et al.* 1986).

Essentially the respondents in diffusion research are asked to recall or remember their own history of adoption of an innovation. This method inevitably suffers from recall inaccuracies and may be largely dependent on the respondent's memory or education, or the length of time since the innovation was adopted, or indeed the salience or obviousness of the innovation. One possible solution to this recall problem is to spend more time on process research and use multiple data-collecting points over a set time period from initial diffusion to the top of the 'S' curve. At each point in time respondents are asked about whether they have adopted and what influenced that decision. A good case in point would be where an industry or employer introduces a no smoking policy: measurements or observations should be made immediately before implementation, during implementation, and immediately after the policy went into effect. Other important steps that could be taken to reduce recall inaccuracy include choosing an innovation that is salient and has been diffused rapidly; pre-testing survey questions and training interviewers; and, third, verifying respondents' recall by using other source data (if available), for example, medical records, newspapers, and other archival records (Rogers 1983).

CONSEQUENTIALISM AND THE PROBLEM OF EQUALITY

Communication of innovation theory was created in Western industrialized societies that subscribed to the idea that technological innovation was 'good' but that it was also the cornerstone to economic and social development. The classical diffusion model, developed in the United States and Europe and based on the Ryan and Gross study, paid little, if any, attention to social structure and the consequential impact of an innovation on a community. Most studies were conducted, as I have attempted to demonstrate, through empirical data-collecting methods that assumed innovation-diffusion was good and progressive, concentrated on adopters, and analysed the means or medium of communication. When the model was adopted by developing countries in the Third World in the 1960s and 1970s researchers began to question this dominant paradigm. These Third World scholars began to question whether the classical diffusion model contributed much to economic and/or social development. The issue, they argued (Diaz-Bordenave 1974), was one not simply of adding structural variables to diffusion analyses but examining innovation-diffusion in the context of a completely different social structure. This viewpoint, accompanied by a theoretical rethinking, led to a paradigm shift in conceptions of development. At the heart of this rethinking was whether technology was the necessary prerequisite for economic development. This paradigm shift in innovation-diffusion modelling mirrors to some extent the paradigm shift discussed in Chapter 1 in relation to health promotion theory. The shift may be illustrated below.

Clearly in this 'new' paradigm greater emphasis was placed on a paced programme of development that was socially and culturally sensitive to local economies, that considered egalitarianism as a central issue, and held developed countries equally to blame for underdevelopment in the Third World.

It produced questions that challenged the classical assumptions associated with innovation-diffusion. These questions centred around the likely consequences of an innovation in terms of employment or unemployment, the equitable distribution of incomes, socio-economic differences, and advantaged and disadvantaged groups. Additionally researchers were

Classical paradigm of development	New paradigm of development
1. Economic growth.	1. Equality of distribution.
2. Capital intensive technology.	2. Improving the quality of life. Emphasis on relevant technology.
3. Centralized planning of development.	3. Self-reliance in development at local level.
4. Mainly internal causes of underdevelopment.	4. Internal *and* external causes of underdevelopment.

Source: Adapted from Rogers 1983

concerned with the movement of migrant labour from the countryside to urban centres as a result of innovations.   They (Beltran 1974; Grunig 1971) began to ask whether the innovation was appropriate for the country's stage of development. Is public welfare at the heart of innovation diffusion or is it more to do with profit motivation for wealthy industrialists? Of course these concerns were voiced largely in response to technological innovations but the 'new' paradigm holds true when examining innovation-diffusion concerned with new public policy, schools curriculum development, or a new immunization programme. The difference is that here the innovation may be less salient to the potential adopters but may have longer-term impact. The kernel in the argument of the researchers developing the 'new' paradigm is that it is the social structure which largely determines the nature and degree of adoption of an innovation rather than the individual characteristics of the adopters. Diffusion strategies need, therefore, to be aware or take account of social structures if development is to be more equitable and the consequences of the innovation-diffusion are desirable.

GENERALIZATIONS

Rogers and Shoemaker (1971) outline 103 generalizations related to the communication of innovations based on research findings over a number of years. Some academics (Downs and Mohr 1976) have questioned the reliability of these diffusion generalizations stating that 'perhaps the most alarming characteristic of the body of empirical study of innovation is the extreme variance among its findings, what we [Downs and Mohr] call instability. . . . this occurs with relentless regularity. One should certainly expect some variation in social science research, but the record in the field of innovation is beyond interpretation. In Rogers and Shoemakers' own evaluation the reliability rates vary from as low as 15–20 per cent to as high as 75–80 per cent.' Four generalizations do score well however and it might be worthwhile examining these briefly before concluding the chapter.

1 The first generalization concerns time and the adoption period. Full diffusion of most major innovations follows the S-shaped diffusion curve as pioneered by Ryan and Gross (1943), and as outlined in Figure 9.2. Diffusion time varies from seven years (adoption of penicillin by physicians) to fifty years (adoption of kindergartens by education authorities in the USA (Yarbrough 1981).

2 The second generalization concerns the rate of adoption and states that the rate of acceptance of an innovation varies according to i) the characteristics of the innovation and ii) the attributes of the individual adoption units (adopter characteristics). Innovations are more rapidly adopted if they are salient and offer a demonstrable advantage over existing practice, if they are easy to understand and use and if they can be used on a trial basis initially. Microwave ovens might be a useful example here. Second, the characteristics of individual adopters demand more attention from communication researchers than all other aspects of diffusion theory put together and so the generalization that the time of adoption by individual adoption units is related to the characteristics of the adoption unit is born out by extensive research. Since the rate of diffusion approximates to a normal distribution curve researchers have separated the diffusion curve into standard deviation units and then examined the characteristics of the individual adopters falling into these five deviation units. The innovators (see p. 190) who comprise the first unit are characteristically venturesome and scientific, have a high educational standard, think abstractly, and tend to be leaders in large organizations. They, unlike the last adopter unit (laggards), are typically more technically competent and have greater wealth but they are unlikely to be opinion leaders in local communities. These are much more likely to be members of the second and third units of adoption, namely early adopters and the early majority respectively.

3 The third generalization concerns the stages adopters go through in the adoption process and it states that several functional stages are involved in the diffusion process by units of adopters. In Rogers and Shoemaker's model these included knowledge, persuasion, decision, and confirmation but could be adapted to allow for a five-stage process (see p. 186). In many ways this generalization is borne out by personal experiences since with any major decision surrounding the take-up of a new idea or product we need to be aware of the innovation, be persuaded by its efficacy/usefulness, make a decision based on this, and adopt.

4 The fourth and final generalization relates to information sources and states that the further down the diffusion curve one goes the more the source of information will change from mass media to interpersonal. Yarbrough and Klongan (1974) found that media sources served only to draw awareness of an innovation to potential adopters and indeed were the most important source of information at the knowledge awareness

stage but during the decision adoption stage slipped to third ranking, as interpersonal contact with peers became much more important. This generalization is perhaps the most contentious and many researchers have questioned it (Coleman *et al.* 1966; Schramm 1977; Maccoby *et al.* 1977). Nevertheless it is important to note that information sources and their impact vary with the type of innovation and the functional stages of adoption.

CONCLUSION

This chapter, although ostensibly concerned with communication theory, has focused on innovation-diffusion. This is for two fundamental reasons. First, innovation-diffusion research and theory is a key, if not the key, to more general communication theory. It is at the heart of the basic model outlined in the first paragraph of the chapter. Without an understanding of how and why new ideas and products are communicated through a community or social system over time, the general body of communication theory would be sadly lacking. Second, work around innovation-diffusion theory allows health promotion specialists to borrow ideas and practices so that programmes, projects, ideas, and policies in health promotion can more easily and readily be diffused and adopted by practitioners. These can be on a large scale like the Stanford and North Karelia programme described in Chapter 2 in this book or they could be on a much more local scale like the introduction of a new teaching pack in a school or the introduction of a 'trim trail' in the local community. As professional researchers often plead that good research can be achieved on a low-budget small-scale project, so innovation theory can be adapted to small, locally based programmes. The theory only provides a framework for practice, or, perhaps more importantly and in keeping with the tone of this book, the practice should inform and mould the theory. As mentioned above, innovation-diffusion theory has undergone a paradigm shift that now allows it to take cognizance of social structure. Practitioners working within that social structure have the opportunity to determine the shape and nature of that shift.

REFERENCES

Basch, C. E., Eveland, J. D., and Portnoy, B. (1986) 'Diffusion systems for education and learning about health', *Family and Community Health* 9(2): 1–26.

Becher, T. and Maclure, S. (1978) *The Politics of Curriculum Change*, London: Hutchinson.

Beltran, L. (1974) 'Rural development and social communication: relationships and strategies', in R. Crawford and W. Ward (eds) *Communication Strategies for Rural Development*, Proceedings of Cornell–CIAT International Symposium.

Brown, L. A. (1981) *Innovation Diffusion – A New Perspective*, London: Methuen.

Caplan, N. and Nelson, S. (1973) 'On being useful: the nature and consequences of psychological research on social problems', *American Psychologist* 28: 199–24.

Coleman, J., Katz, E., and Menzel, H. (1966) *Medical Innovation: A Diffusion Study*, New York: Bobbs-Merrill.

DeFleur, M. and Ball-Rokeach, S. (1975) *Theories of Mass Communication*, New York: David McKay.

Diaz–Bordenave, J. (1974) 'Communication and adoption of agricultural innovation in Latin America', in R. Crawford and W. Ward (eds) *Communication Strategies for Rural Development*, Proceedings of Cornell–CIAT International Symposium.

Downs, G. and Mohr, L. (1976) 'Conceptual issues in the study of innovation', *Administrative Science Quarterly* 21: 700–14.

Fliegel F. (1966) 'Attributes of innovations as factors in diffusion', *American Journal of Sociology* 72: 235–48.

Green, L. W. and Lewis, F. M. (1986) *Measurement and Evaluation in Health Education and Health Promotion*, Palo Alto, CA: Mayfield.

Grunig, J. (1971) 'Communication and the economic decision-making processes of Columbian peasants', *Economic Development and Cultural Change* 19: 580–97.

Hannon, P. J. and Zucker, D. M. (1989) 'Analysis issues in school-based health promotion studies', *Health Education Quarterly* 16(2): 315–20.

Havelock, R. (1974) *Educational Innovation in the United States*, Vol. 1, University of Michigan Report.

Hovland, C. and Janis, I. (1959) *Personality & Persuasibility*, New Haven, CT: Yale University Press.

Lazarsfeld, P. (1963) 'Mass media and personal influence', in W. Schramm, (ed.) *The Science of Communication* New York: Basic Books.

Ledwith, F. and Peers, I. (1988) *Development and National Dissemination of Smoking Education of Schools*, University of Manchester (unpublished).

Lipstein, B. and McGuire, W. (1978) *Evaluating Advertising: A Bibliography of the Communications Process*, New York: Advertising Research Foundation.

Maccoby, N., Farquhar, J. W., Wood, P. D., and Alexander, J. K. (1977) 'Reducing the risk of cardiovascular disease effects of a community-based campaign on knowledge and behaviour', *Journal of Community Health* 3: 100–14.

Macdonald, G. (1986) 'Participation is the best form of learning', *Journal of Health at School* 2: 3.

McGuire W. (1978) in *Evaluating Advertising: A Bibliography of the Communications Process*, New York: Advertising Research Foundation.

Newman, R. and Nutbeam, D. (1989) 'The Family Smoking Education Project: What do teachers think of it?', *Health Education Journal* 48: 9–14.

Nutbeam, D., Smith, C., and Catford, J. (1990) 'Evaluation in health education: a review of progress, possibilities and problems', *Journal of Epidemiology and Community Health* 44: 83–9.

Parcel, G. *et al.* (1989) 'Translating theory into practice: intervention strategies for the diffusion of a health promotion innovation', *Family and Community Health* 12(3): 1–13.

Portnoy, B. Anderson, D. M., and Eriksen, M. (1989) 'Application of diffusion theory to health promotion research', *Family and Community Health* 12(3): 63–71.

Puska, P., Nissinen, A., Tuomilehto, J. *et al.* (1985) 'The community based strategy to prevent coronary heart disease: conclusions from ten years of the Karelia Project', *Annual Review of Public Health* 6: 147–63.

Robertson, T. S. (1971) *Innovative Behaviour and Communications*, New York: Holt, Rinehart & Winston.

Rogers, E. (1983) *Diffusion of Innovations*, New York: The Free Press, Macmillan.

Rogers, E. *et al.* (1970) *Diffusion of Innovations in Brazil, Nigeria and India*, Michigan State University Research Report No. 24.

Rogers, E. M. and Shoemaker, F. F. (1971) *Communication of Innovations: A Cross-cultural Approach*, New York: The Free Press.

Roling, N. *et al.* (1976) 'The diffusion of innovations and the issue of equity in rural development', *Communication Research* 3: 155–70.

Ryan, B. and Gross, N. C. (1943) 'The diffusion of hybrid seed corn in two Iowa communities', *Rural Sociology* 8: 15–24.

Schramm, W. (1977) *Big Media, Little Media: Tools and Technology for Instruction*, London: Sage.

Schramm, W. and Lerner, D. (eds) (1978) *Communication and Change: The Last Ten Years – and the Next*, Honolulu: University Press of Hawaii.

TACADE (1986) *Monitor* 3(1).

Tarde, G. (1903) *The Laws of Imitation*, New York: Holt.

Yarbrough, P. (1981) 'Communication theory and nutrition education research', *Journal of Nutrition Education* 13(1): 16–26.

Yarbrough, P. and Klongan, G. (1974) *Adoption and Diffusion of Innovations – Research Findings in Community Dental Health – Organising for Action*, Sociology Report No. 113, Iowa State University.

Yarbrough, P., Klonglan, G., and Lutz, G. (1970) *System and Personal Variables as Predictors of Individual Adoption of Behaviour*, Sociology Report No. 86, Iowa State University.

Chapter 10

The growth of health promotion theory and its rational reconstruction

Lessons from the philosophy of science

Don Rawson

CONFIDENCE AND CRISES IN HEALTH PROMOTION

As health promotion work has expanded in recent years so the accepted prescriptions for appraising health science and evaluating health interventions have proved to be inadequate. Theorists have either tended to search other disciplines for a scientific basis to their work (witness this volume) or else have concentrated on expounding the ideological basis of health promotion (compare, for example, the anthology in Rodmell and Watts 1986). Neither approach, however, has led to the creation of a corpus of knowledge particular to health promotion or to a coherent set of methods worthy of discipline status.

Is there a paradigm shift from health education to health promotion?

Since the 1970s the efforts of health educators have come under increasing criticism. (Contrast the vast array of critical evaluations from differing perspectives all summating into a disenchantment with the panacea health education had originally promised: Adams 1985; Bowman 1976; Dwore and Matarazzo 1981; Labonte and Penfold 1981; Neutens 1984; Tones 1983; Tones *et al.* 1990; Whitehead 1989; Williams and Aspin 1980.)

There has been at least a crisis of spirit as critics from a variety of perspectives have highlighted the relative ineffectiveness of health education campaigns which are focused on changing health lifestyles. Added to this are the overwhelmingly daunting problems of attempting to achieve major health reforms in the existing social and political order.

Whether or not the very foundations of health education have been shaken, the criticisms illustrate the cramped and teetering structure of a subject built on unsound philosophical grounds. Whether or not health education and health promotion can be regarded as possessing a scientific basis, the continuing growth of criticism suggests it will be necessary to become increasingly conversant with the kind of issues addressed by the philosophy of science: namely, elucidation of the essential nature of the subject, characterization of progress and growth, and questioning of the basis of its authority.

Champions of the self-styled new health promotion movement in public health have been vociferous in proclaiming a paradigm shift from the old health education to health promotion. Although there has been dissatisfaction with some health education work, is this the same as a transfer of allegiance to a new paradigm?

Thomas Kuhn's (1957, 1962) descriptions of scientific revolutions as paradigm shifts has been broadly welcomed as an explanation of the displacement and progression of ideas within disciplines. Kuhn argues that paradigm shifts take place as social movements in the scientific community, with researchers abandoning orthodox theories and methods (or paradigms) when a new paradigm is seen to assimilate or go beyond the older established one.

In just such a manner, it is said, the term health promotion appeared more or less abruptly during the 1980s and rapidly achieved a fashionable status. Many professionals who ten years ago were engaged in the development of health education now appear to align themselves with the new health promotion movement.

The distinction between health education and health promotion has, however, been both contentious and confused (Tones 1986). Recently, some consensus has begun to emerge, redefining health education almost exclusively in terms of individually focused campaigns designed to change health lifestyles (WHO 1984). As health promotion gains ground, health education is increasingly faced with a crisis of legitimacy. Where health education is identified solely with the attempt to change individual lifestyles it is also regarded as synonymous with victim blaming (Crawford 1977; Labonte and Penfold 1981).

Prior to the advent of health promotion, however, health educationalists had already begun to define the parameters of health education more widely to include consideration of structural features and advocacy of social reform (Anderson 1980; Crawford 1977; Draper et al. 1979; Thorpe 1982). In Britain at least, the proliferation and dissemination of hypothetical health education models during the 1980s facilitated a reconsideration of the appropriate aims and methods of health education. It may be that such collections of models are now more appropriately described as health promotion taxonomies, containing health education models.

Described in this way, the change to health promotion resembles a paradigm shift. Kuhn's analysis relies, though, on the scientists' ability to recognize truth (or at least the prospects of a going concern). As Kuhn (1970) expresses it, 'Scientific knowledge, like language, is intrinsically the common property of the group or else nothing at all.' Lakatos (1970), though, critizes Kuhn's account as being little more than 'mob science', that is, scientific progress determined through consensus in the scientific élite.

The implication is that, although Kuhn suggests the new scientific paradigm has greater theoretical content than its predecessor (that is, it explains the world better), Kuhn's analysis excludes the possibility of a rational and normative means of appraising scientific growth.

In recent years Kuhn's work has suffered a declining influence amongst philosophers of science, partly because the historiographical basis is regarded as too simplistic. The idea of cycles between normal and revolutionary science has in particular been difficult to sustain. The epistemological basis to Kuhn's work has also received considerable criticism. Chalmers (1976) claims that Kuhn's popularity is undeserved and that he conflates three distinct views: subjectivist, consensual, and objectivist. Although Kuhn argues for elements of all three, Chalmers points out that ultimately Kuhn chooses the consensual criteria for appraising science.

Was the change to health promotion purely a social movement in the occupations of health education or has it entailed real changes in professional thinking and practice? Although many have adopted the health promotion rubric there is some doubt that it has been accompanied by changes in substance. In a nationwide study of the training and development needs of British health education officers, Rawson and Grigg (1988) were unable to locate any factors which reliably differentiated the work of those involved in health education as opposed to health promotion. Numerous health education organizations, moreover, are staffed by health promotion officers and likewise, some health promotion units are run by specialists with a health education title.

Another critical review of recent changes in public health policy similarly concludes, 'Health promotion to date has either comprised the strategies of health education under a new name or has consisted of much rhetoric and little action' (Research Unit in Health & Behavioural Change, University of Edinburgh 1989). In short, there appears to be more of a shift in title than a true shift of paradigms. In the occupations of health education the change of label to health promotion may none the less be welcomed as an opportunity to declare anew the purposes of an emerging profession.

Most writers now appear to have accepted that health education is redefined as a part of a broader health promotion perspective. It is to be hoped that the sudden professional exodus to health promotion does not in the end signal the complete abandonment of health education or replace one practice having an inadequate theoretical basis with another equally inadequate thesis bereft of epistemological foundations.

THE PHILOSOPHY OF SCIENTIFIC METHOD

As with all disciplines, the philosophy of scientific method is best characterized through the approach it takes to defining problems rather than by
the current content of its subject matter.

Interestingly, Gellner (1974) contends that the philosophy of science has
also been working through a crisis of legitimacy. Like politics generally, he
argues, it fluctuates between poles of liberalism and authoritarianism. The
first tries to protect science from the arbitrary limits imposed by authority
which ultimately lead to scientific stagnation. The second attempts to protect
science from stultification brought through the chaos of anarchy. Gellner
goes on to identify two corresponding modes of resolving the crisis. One
is to invoke something bigger than all of us, something, that is, objective.
The alternative means of validation is to believe only in our own internal
premises, resulting in something relative and subjective. Whatever scientists
are, or do, supplies this agnostic and anthropocentric solution.

For Gellner, theories take on a political force with the movement from
one pole to the other. In the struggle for scientific survival, it is necessary
to discover how and why one theory comes to be regarded as more scientific
or true than another. In the parlance of the philosophy of science a *universal
demarcation criterion* is created (Popper 1959, 1963).

The philosophy of scientific method then directs us to appraise theories
in the light of the generalized demarcation problem. This consists of asking
how true science can be differentiated from pseudo- or non-science, and
how rival theoretical accounts of the same subject matter can be reconciled.
Translated to the field of health promotion the problem is to distinguish
true or 'authentic' health promotion from other promotions of health (say,
for example, commercial advertising which incorporates a pseudo 'health'
message to motivate product buying). For public credibility to be maintained
there is a pressing need to establish a clear demarcation criterion. Within the
professional field there is no less urgent a problem of differentiating health
educational from wider health promotional activity and of establishing the
relative effectiveness of different approaches. If health promotion theory
continues to develop it will become increasingly necessary to address the
generalized demarcation problem.

The philosophy of scientific method approaches the demarcation problem
through two complementary paths: by elucidating the epistemological basis
of scientific method and by historiographical reconstructions of scientific
progress. Theorists, though, have been slow to journey along either route
in their discussions of health promotion.

THE NEED FOR EPISTEMOLOGY

Understanding human knowledge is more than a paradox. More than the vain pursuit of armchair philosophers, it is ultimately our only touchstone of truth. But to say that the shape of all knowledge is guided by our view of what knowledge is or should be is, of course, a mere metaphysical adage. And, like most well-worn issues, its significance declines over time. The original puzzle of understanding knowledge which so preoccupies philosophers can come to be seen as an impossible and largely irrelevant quandary. After all, it might be said, what point is there in procrastinating about such intangibles when there are real and practical issues to solve? More strongly, the same notion, that there are certain irreducible aspects of human existence, can be taken as a justification for activism, the ideology which opposes any kind of complacency, including theorizing (Popper 1957). Within health promotion some who advocate radical action are also intolerant of theory work. Equally, pragmatists who resist intellectual activity see philosophizing as irrelevant or misleading (e.g. Seymour 1984).

Even scientists sometimes show little patience with problems of epistemology. In trying to expand their body of systematic knowledge they focus only upon specific problems related to their discipline. Now scientists can, and some do, practise successful science without an explicit formulation of the epistemological assumptions underlying their methods. Claiming to hold no specific philosophy, however, is at best a pretence. Perhaps of greatest consequence, implicit epistemologies are more difficult to criticize, and therefore improve, than are explicit ideas. Epistemology is in this sense unavoidable. As Rosenberg (1988) aptly describes, 'Even the claim that philosophical reflection is irrelevant to advancing knowledge ... is itself a philosophical claim.'

SOME HISTORIOGRAPHICAL CONSIDERATIONS

The models of health education debate

During the last decade health education (in Great Britain anyway) has been awash with debate about appropriate health education models. The subject frequently surfaces at conferences and has been carried along with the ebb and flow of journal correspondence. The professional field has expressed and continues to express concern with the appropriate selection of working models. (See, for example, the issue of the *Health Education Journal*, Vol. 49, 1990, devoted to theoretical debate.)

Health education models are hypothesized to be coherent approaches to health education practice, such as the 'self-empowerment model' or the 'social action model'. They are considered to embody different concepts of health and education, diverse methodologies and means of evaluation, and consequently different repertoires of knowledge and skills from practitioners. Most significantly, they have been generated, almost entirely, from within the practice field. In this sense, models of health education represent the most likely source for developing a body of knowledge particular to health promotion. They may be distinguished completely from explanatory models imported from other disciplines (e.g. the health belief model), though this has also been a major concern to some theorists in health promotion (see, for example, Catford and Parish 1989; Downie *et al*. 1990; Tones *et al*. 1990; Research Unit in Health & Behavioural Change, University of Edinburgh 1989).

From the models debate *within* health education, however, Rawson and Grigg (1988) identified seventeen published taxonomies or collections of health education models in Britain alone. Many of the taxonomies are only sketchiliy described in one- or two-page articles or have gone no further than brief presentations at professional conferences. One notable account has managed strongly to influence a generation of health education specialists whilst remaining largely absent from the usual channels of academic publication (Beattie 1980, 1984, 1991). The content of taxonomies ranges from simplistic linguistic juggling (e.g. Tannahill 1985) to complex structuralist arguments (e.g. Dorn 1983). Recent additions to the burgeoning catalogue of models include a health promotion model by Catford and Parish (1989), three historical 'approaches' to health education by Downie *et al*. (1990), interpretations of the Burrell and Morgan scheme (1985) by Caplan and Holland (1990) and Taylor (1990), plus a revision of the French and Adams taxonomy (1986) by French (1990).

The continuing proliferaton of models shows no sign of abating and brings the number of taxonomies to over a score. Strangely, most of the model makers seem to be unaware of the existence of each other's efforts. At least there is little cross-referencing with either critical appraisal or cumulative building of ideas. Generally, it appears that the taxonomies are produced from first principles, in order to explain some particular health education initiative or in order to set out the range of possible approaches to health education activity for different professional groups who have discovered a core health promotion role. The plurality of efforts leads inevitably to much redundancy and slow, if not retarded, theoretical growth. Whilst the expression of more models may testify to persistent underlying theoretical issues, there is also the real possibility of theoretical fragmentation and practical confusion with well over 100 resultant models to choose from.

Unfortunately there has been very little in the way of either analytical or empirical research to test the validity of the putative health education models. Collins (1982, 1984) explored the ramifications of different practice models across four professional groups using so-called illuminative methodologies. Nutbeam (1984) also investigated the health education models held by different professional groups, using a different but limited methodology. The samples were also respectively very small and eccentric, however, making generalization difficult.

In a more extensive empirical study Rawson and Grigg (1988) surveyed the health education models preferred by over 100 health education officers plus a similar number of their role partners and set these against actual records of health education activities. The methodology made innovative use of an interactive computer program (MODEFI or MOdels DEFinition Instrument). This locates individual or group preferences against a set of well-known taxonomies (Beattie 1980; Draper 1983; Ewles and Simnett 1985; Tones 1981). Factor analysis revealed that the nineteen separate models generated from the principal taxonomies represented could be subsumed in a spectrum of seven meta models. In all, the results showed that the occupational philosophy of health education officers could be characterized as a preference for working through intermediaries such as other health professionals and lay workers, rather than through direct appeals to at-risk groups. The role partners, however, saw health education work as influencing public health through more direct and less catalytic approaches. More than this, the health education specialists showed a marked concern with methodologies of facilitating rather than disseminating health education content.

Similar names are invoked by many of the model makers for their various models. French (1984) analyses several of the taxonomies and attempts to reduce the surfeit by identifying areas of linguistic overlap. French shows that many of the same themes are indeed reiterated, suggesting some theoretical unity and redundancy of effort. Closer analysis, however, also reveals that the same labels sometimes conceal quite distinct concepts. For example, Ewles and Simnett (1985) and Tones (1981) both describe an educational approach as a distinct model of health education. Ewles and Simnett say it aims to equip individuals with the knowledge and understanding for rational decision making about health issues. Appropriate health education is said to address the causes and effects of health and illness and may include an exploration of values and attitudes. They also specify, however, that the educational approach should inform but not influence. As they express it, 'Information about health is presented in as value-free a way as possible.'

Tones, in contrast, is critical of education based on the supposition that facts can be presented from a neutral position for people to make an untethered rational choice. Instead he advocates a sophisticated version of the educational model which recognizes the need to explore beliefs, clarify values, and give practice in decision making. Indeed, the concept of informed choice is central to any educational model but also implies inescapable assumptions about freedom of choice. As Tones (1981) cogently states, 'For many individuals the options are limited or non-existent.'

It is also relevant to note that, in countries where health education exists as an established academic subject, models' debates concerning the essential nature of health education have had little showing. In the United States, attention has largely focused on the appropriate role and function of health educators. This has tended to be both prescriptive and atheoretical, however, lacking process indications and making naive assumptions about the unity of purpose (Bowman 1976; Galli 1978). Neutens (1984) argues for further role delineation research as a means of establishing a unifying philosophy. Similarly, in the Netherlands, there has been a primary concern with role composition (Krijnen *et al*. 1982).

The relationship of models, taxonomies, and theories

Within the philosophy of science generally, models appear to be regarded unproblematically, and are usually described as preliminary or temporary devices to assist the scientists' thinking rather than as logically necessary components of theory building. Lakatos (1970), for example, says, 'A model is a set of initial conditions (possibly together with some of the observational theories) which one knows is bound to be replaced during further development of the [research] programme.' Nagel (1961) gives a stronger role to models for fleshing out the logical skeleton of a theories explanatory structure which he says is often in visualizable terms. That is, models make the theory concrete. Theories, in Nagel's view, cannot provide adequate explanation without models. In the social sciences a similar notion to Nagel's can be found in Blalock (1971) who argues that models enable a transition from the verbal form of theories to more precise research techniques. Mathematical formulations in particular, Blalock sees as helping 'recast' verbal theories as testable models. This insight has a special relevance for health promotion which continues to thrive in a mostly oral tradition. Major developments in practice tend to be told narratively at conferences rather than being documented in theoretical literature.

It is pertinent to ask whether health education models are necessary components of theoretical development or whether they should be regarded as temporary constructions in the development of health promotion theory.

French and Adams (1986) envisage a construction sequence from laying the foundations in ideology, through theory building, to the development of models. That is, models are regarded as the end product of health promotion philosophy. They function to support practice through identifying goals and shaping strategies.

For the most part, however, health promotion taxonomies can be seen to have developed in the opposite direction. At least, the greater abundance of models which have appeared have been unaccompanied by much detailed theory work or explicit ideology.

Models, moreover, are seldom followed through. At a descriptive level the models' wider and more extensive implications are excluded. The often-criticized medical model, for example, is seldom explored as a basis of appropriate intervention by medical professionals. As a normative (ideal) account the underlying theory receives only the crudest analysis. The educational model, for example, has little correspondence with the educational issues emphasized by educationalists (cf. Dearden 1972; Hirst 1983; Peters 1977).

Rather, health education models appear at first sight to be as much about forms of service delivery available to health education specialists as about health education principles. That is, the models may conflate role boundaries with health promotion principles. In describing the educational model, for example, are the models not describing the deployment of skills by practitioners from an educational background rather than unfolding an approach based on educational principles? Downie et al. (1990) are critical of the models debate on precisely these grounds. They see the putative models as misleading and oversimplified viewpoints detracting from interprofessional collaboration. Downie et al, however, miss the epistemological point. They are mistaken to assume the models debate is only a reflection of professional rivalry. Rather, it is a manifestation of an emerging profession's struggle to develop core theoretical underpinnings from the practice base. What is required in health promotion, as in any other emerging occupation, is a new epistemology of practice (Schön 1983). That is, a means of distinguishing and codifying the essential operating characteristics of practice and of articulating the development of goals.

Iconic and analogic models in health promotion

Diesing (1971) lists eight separate usages of the term 'models' and cautions that the terms 'model' and 'theory' are often loosely employed and sometimes reversed in meaning. Warr (1980) provides a most useful summary of the function of models generally and notes that the term contains a confused collection of meanings. He also points out that various reviewers have been dismayed at the disparate variety of meanings and lack of theoretical integretion. For Warr, however, models are separate from conceptual frameworks, paradigms, and theories. Although the language varies considerably, most contributors to thinking about the epistemological status of models typically differentiate two types of models, which Warr, somewhat prosaically refers to as Models 1 and 2. More lucidly, they are iconic or analogic representations. The first are simplified descriptions of some aspect of known reality, portraying a literal or isomorphic image of nature. The second are analogies or metaphors used to assist our understanding about nature and may have no direct counterpart in reality.

Although the term 'approaches' is preferred by Ewles and Simnett (1985), their taxonomy contains five detailed iconic models. In addition to descriptive accounts of each model they also supply examples of the application of each approach in practice along with the aim and appropriate health education activity for each model.

Model systems in health promotion which are predominantly iconic, such as the Ewles and Simnett taxonomy, have the advantage of being limited to that which is currently observable. By simplifying the reality of practice they also help reduce the complexities of health promotion to manageable proportions. This makes them readily believable and attractive to those who eschew intellectual work. Being tied to the here and now, however, means that they have limited generalizability and cannot be easily adapted to changes. In the world of health, of course, change is the one certainty.

Iconic models in the final analysis reduce to operational definitions. Health promotion comes to be defined as what health promoters do. As Tones (1981) warns, however, this is fraught with the same difficulties and circularity of reasoning as are other operational definitions (like intelligence being what intelligence tests measure). Effective and appropriate health promotion could instead be that which no one has yet developed. In the absence of any higher order theory showing how the various models are integrated to the same overall purpose there is also the constant danger of contradictory practice. Different health education models may cancel out the achievements of other approaches through mutually contradictory efforts. Theoretical growth at a practical level is thus essential to the development of coherent strategy.

Beattie's (1980, 1984, 1991) account of health education and health promotion offers in contrast a strongly analogic taxonomy. The work partly grew out of Bernstein's (1980) concepts of codes and control and makes use of the cross-classification scheme proposed by C. Wright Mills (1959). It thus stands on a firm theoretical footing. The resulting repertoire is drawn from the attempt to combine models of health with models of education. Two intersecting axes, which are claimed to be fundamental dimensions of health education, create a 'structural map' of the possible range of health promotion models.

Analogic taxonomies such as Beattie's, in contrast to iconic representations, can assimilate changes since the theoretical structure already contains the relationships and progressions between elements. They may even extend the possibilities of practice by indicating a form of health promotion which as yet has to be attempted.

The disadvantage of analogic systems is that they may be seen as remote from the detail of reality and so of limited help in dealing with the concrete issues encountered in practice. That is, the theoretical abstraction may require further translation to be of immediate benefit.

Caplan and Holland (1990), French and Adams (1986), and Tannahill (1985), amongst others, describe their sets of models as typologies. Typological systems, however, are more usually taken to refer to a dimensional classification, which means a continuously graded sequence of elements with labels attached to the extremes or poles (e.g. introvert–extravert).

Although some of the collections of models are claimed to be dimensional (e.g. Beattie 1991; Caplan and Holland 1990; Nutbeam 1984) none actually treats the variety of models in this way. Mid-points on the dimensions are not considered, neither are progressions along the continua referred to in anything other than a cursory manner. Consequently, it would be more internally consistent if the intersecting axes of these systems were redrawn to recast the models as nominal categories.

There is, coincidentally, another sense in which taxonomies may be the more appropriate form of categorization. It is interesting to recall that much of evolutionary theory was propagated in the soil of taxonomic development. Darwin's work made essential use of the systematic collections of fossils and animal specimens catalogued by early naturalists who painstakingly assembled taxonomies of species. Regarded in this way, health promotion taxonomies may be best regarded as embryonic formulations necessarily preceding the maturation of theory.

The search for models has, however, been condemned by Kelvin (1980) who sees it as being empty. As he expresses it, 'To think of models is primitive. We should look for the phenomena for which we have to account.' Restated, there is a possible tautology in explaining the functioning of health promotion through modelling health education work. Can a part be used to explain the whole?

Suppe (1977) also criticizes the idea that models are essential explanations and cites quantum mechanics as an example of theory work not dependent upon models. Instead, Suppe contends that models may be heuristically fruitful but not necessary as integral components of theoretical development. For health promotion, however, model construction appears to be the only basis of core theoretical development thus far.

The models debate has unfortunately been limited mostly to discussion of models *within* taxonomies. What is required, however, is debate *between* taxonomies with an attempt to explicate the underlying theoretical principles. Further production of yet more taxonomies which only superficially describe health education and health promotion approaches will not of itself lead to theory development. Instead, health promotion theory should be directed at discovering what characterizes health promotion as opposed to any other subject matter. This should include an analysis of both content and methods. The philosophy of science may assist in this regard by extending the analysis of solutions given to the generalized demarcation problem.

In mainstream philosophy of science, the iconic–analogic distinction has a parallel in the epistemological status of theories. Controversies over the realist or instrumentalist nature of science have come to be redefined instead as debates over the generalized demarcation problem.

ESSENTIALS OF HEALTH PROMOTION

The nature of health and its attainment

The content of health promotion taxonomies is in part predicated upon alternative definitions of health. Health educationalists have long been outspoken in challenging the received notion of health as absence of illness and disease. Birn and Birn (1985) best characterize the prevailing bio-medical concept of health as a defect-apparatus. This means that disease and progressive failure of function are seen as inevitable features of life. Consequently, appropriate health promotion consists of timely screening and other interventions to reduce defects and minimize damage. Instead, Birn and Birn urge a complete move by health educators to a social-medical model emphasizing well-being.

From a wider cultural perspective, Burkitt (1983) has similarly challenged the fact that the Western medical model still dominates health education with an inappropriate basis for understanding health. The WHO concept of Health For All is unlikely to be obtained, moreover, as long as health is defined in terms of illness avoidance. Instead, Burkitt advocates a concept of positive health similar to that found in traditional Chinese medicine.

Downie *et al.* (1990) dispute the implied continuum from negative to positive health and suggest instead that the two concepts are independent. With this orthogonal relationship of concepts it would be possible to be in a state of illness and yet have a state of well-being. Equally, one might have a complete absence of illness but not experience well-being. Positive health, moreover, is said to be a broader concept, embracing well-being, fitness, and other related features (such as balance of physical, mental, and social elements). This analysis offers interesting possibilities for the development of health promotion to integrate with other forms of health intervention. At the very least it represents a move away from the dichotomized impasse between medical and health education ideologies.

Seedhouse (1986) takes a more pluralist view and argues that health is intrinsically composed of multiple meanings and definitions, being both a means and an end in itself. Consequently, he urges health promoters to adopt a fuzzy view of health as a potential, given definition by the wider personal and social context.

Whatever definition of health gains precedence, health is likely to remain an essentially contested concept for health promotion (Gallie 1956). How the issue is debated, more than the resolution of an agreed upon meaning, will in the end dictate whether or not health promotion achieves discipline status.

Another set of epistemic assumptions underlying different approaches to health promotion engenders levels of potential health attainment. That is, a set of expectations about what in principle can be achieved through health promotion. These range from superficial health (which merely keeps illness at bay) through to complete or absolute health (where health is a positive state). Seedhouse (1986) comes nearest to this understanding by distinguishing questions which address 'what is health?' from those which ask 'how can it be achieved?'.

Both Seedhouse (1986) and Downie et al. (1990) make a strong case for health outcomes to be regarded as relative. The achievement of absolute health (as in the WHO's declaration of Health For All) is portrayed as Utopian. Not only are such goals considered to be unrealistic, but, they also imply fundamentally different strategies for health promotion methodology. Appropriate research and evaluation in health promotion would also need to focus on different health outcomes. Assessing relative health improvement requires different states of evidence than the measuring rod of absolute health.

As with all disciplines, health promotion can be best understood by the approaches it takes to solve such problems, rather than by the current nature of the subject matter. In any case, today's health topics will inevitably be replaced by other demands as the world of health continues to change. How well health promotion adapts to change and survives as a discipline will depend upon how efficient its methodologies are. In this sense the putative models or approaches epitomize the essential nature of the emerging discipline. They contain the special characteristics which distinguish health promotion from other subjects. Models debates then are disputes over the appropriate basis for the discipline. That is, they offer different solutions to the generalized demarcation problem in health promotion.

POSSIBLE SOLUTIONS TO THE GENERALIZED DEMARCATION PROBLEM IN HEALTH PROMOTION

The models question can be most usefully explored through a critical appraisal of the various solutions implied in the health promotion taxonomies. Revealing parallels may be drawn between solutions to the demarcation problem in the philosophy of science and the epistemic basis of health promotion theory. Three kinds of solution may be outlined:

1   that only one criterion is acceptable for promoting health (fundamentalist health promotion);
2   that no universal criterion is possible but some solution is possible (evolutionary health promotion);
3   that no criterion is possible, hence all versions are equally acceptable (eclectic health promotion).

Fundamentalist health promotion

Health promotion based on fundamentalist principles sections the world of health initiatives into the total range of possibilities and admits of only one universal criterion for deciding which course to adopt. Other approaches are seen as either irrelevant, misleading (drawing attention away from the 'true causes' of health problems), or, worse, as contradictory (simply adding to the problem). Freudenberg (1978), for example, contends that individually based health education programmes have signally failed to make any impact on public health. The only viable alternative, he insists, is collective action designed to alter the environment thereby facilitating lifestyle changes. Freudenberg also adds, however, that health professionals might resist this advocacy approach, not least because the politicization of their official role would expose them to the risk of censure from their employers.

The current vogue, however, is to make health promotion work community based (Hatch and Kickbusch 1984: Smithies and Adams 1990; Thomas 1983). Indeed, in Britain, a community development approach appears to be recognized as the most 'authentic' or ideal form of practice for health education specialists (Rawson and Grigg 1988).

Community development, however, can mean anything from attempts to change the lifestyle of communities, perhaps appropriately conceived of as a pluralistic version of individual health education (Puska et al. 1983), to the radical use of community empowerment as a vehicle for wider social and political reform (Freire 1972). Whilst community health promotion work offers a constructive possibility for improving public health, there is also a counterpart tendency to insert the term 'community' as a self-justifying prefix to any new health initiative.

Despite the radical politics implied by the health promotion examples, the underlying epistemology corresponds to the solution given by 'militant' positivism familiar to philosophers of science. In essence this led to a demand that all scientific statements be ultimately reducible to some verifiable observation. This form of scientific empiricism dominated the philosophy of science for nearly half of this century. The received view, as Suppe (1977) labels it, set limits on the basic framework for analysing problems in scientific method. This solution gave the sharpest cutting edge to the demarcation criteria but also perpetuated a narrow view of what constitutes scientific knowledge. In their haste to gain scientific respectability, social scientists, for example, tied themselves to the same sinking philosophical ship (Armistead 1974; Harré 1979).

The parallel for health promotion might be that acceptability comes to be synonymous with a demand for all health promotion statements to be ultimately reducible to social policy. Tones (1990) makes a similar point and urges that individualist health education approaches be regarded as complementary to structuralist (or non individualist) health promotion rather than being disgarded as non-acceptable approaches.

Evolutionary health promotion

With this criterion health promotion might be seen as an outgrowth or logical progression of health education. The development of Tones' taxonomy (1981, 1983, 1985, 1986) best illustrates this solution. Health education models are depicted as progressive adaptations to the changing social climate and as a means of survival in the face of governmental health policies. Tones' work originally described a fourfold taxonomy of health education, but has since expanded to incorporate at least five distinct models and to redefine health education as a part of health promotion. Tones also attempts to delineate central and peripheral influences in the wider social and political context.

Several health education taxonomies invoke principles of hierarchical progression or other developmental sequences amongst models. Slavin and Chapman (1985), for example, postulate a developmental progression for both professionals and clients away from the inhibiting strictures set into the health establishment. Seedhouse (1986) also makes the point that health promotion should achieve some level of health in the health promoters. The reflexivity of health promotion is a further epistemological demand hitherto given little consideration in health promotion taxonomies. Perhaps like charity, health promotion should begin at home.

French and Adams (1986) advance a 'tri-phasic' map of health education models. The ordering also reflects the potential and significance for achieving changes in health. The taxonomy includes the corresponding aim, models of health and education along with underlying models of humanity and society for each of the three phases. The hierarchical progression reflects a sequential change or an evolution of health education strategies towards greater health effectiveness.

An evolutionary view of knowledge and scientific progress is mostly associated with Popper (1963) who argues that falsification could be used as a demarcation criterion between science and pseudo- or non-science. The falsificationist demands that all scientific theories should be capable of potential falsification. This means that all theories should be testable or refutable in principle. Popper sees science progressing through a cumulative process of conjectures and refutations in which weaker theories are eliminated and replaced by more powerful versions with increasing empirical verisimilitude (a closer correspondence with reality).

Developmental sequences in taxonomies of health education similarly imply a principle of *increasing health verisimilitude*. That is, succeeding or higher models in the sequence are considered to be more effective in realizing health benefits. Typically this has been associated with a greater emphasis on structural changes. Conversely, health education models further down the sequence are more likely to be associated with falsifications or failures to bring about health benefits. Any paradigm shift from health education to health promotion may be best understood in this light.

According to the Duhem-Quine thesis, however, theories can be rescued from falsification simply by a relevant adjustment to the background knowledge. The problem is to locate which components are refuted and which are to be retained. With health promotion it is similarly important to discover at what point health education initiatives cease to be effective or what aspect of different approaches may be modified to better suit the aims of health promotion.

Eclectic health promotion

This position is based on the principle that all approaches to health promotion are equally plausible, since no one criterion is possible. The selection of appropriate activity is therefore based either on pragmatic considerations or is arbitrary and random. The Ewles and Simnett (1985) taxonomy, for example, makes explicit the eclectic nature of health promotion work. As they expound, 'In our view there is no-one "right" approach to health education'. Whilst this may be viewed charitably as a liberal solution, in which choice is left to the sagacity of the practitioner, it amounts to an epistemologically arbitrary or anarchic solution. It may seem surprising to equate Ewles and Simnett's otherwise conservative work with epistemological anarchism. Of course their formulation was not intended that way. The epistemic basis of their work none the less implies such a solution by default, as does any pragmatist taxonomy offering no objective rationale for the selection of appropriate health promotion methodologies (cf. Catford and Parish 1989; Downie et al. 1990).

Beyond this, such approaches foresee neither contradictions nor professional dilemmas in choosing one model over another or electing any combination of models. The alternative interpretation is to see the health educator exercising choice as also exercising a form of élitism (which means a return to fundamentalist health promotion).

Within the philosophy of science, Feyerabend's thesis (1975) advocates an extreme form of relativism. A resolute anarchist and Dadaist, Feyerabend argues that all theories are equally right or wrong and therefore equally acceptable or rejectable. Originally a stout hearted Popperian, Feyerabend has since challenged all rational normative solutions to the generalized demarcation problem, contending that, if applied, they would have the effect of shackling scientific progress. Lakatos (1970), however, argues that unless we are to create a situation of real anarchism (where pseudoscience has equal status with true science) there is a need for a rational and conventional solution. But, Feyerabend insists, all rational alternatives are founded on unrealistic assumptions about epistemological commensurability of theories. Rather, he sees knowledge growing in an ocean of incompatible ideas. Epistemological anarchism, therefore, is offered as the only tenable solution.

Within health promotion, a number of theorists reach conclusions carrying the same epistemic implications. In filling out their 'choice-change-champion' framework, Catford and Parish (1989) present a highly eclectic battery of imported models to guide health promotion. Their selection ranges from social learning theory (Bandura 1977) with its emphasis on self-efficacy to social marketing (Manoff 1985). Whilst such models are arguably contradictory, the Catford and Parish framework treats them as totally discrete influences at different and apparently unrelated stages in the overall framework of health promotion. The theoretical influences, that is, are regarded as incommensurable. No linking mechanisms are hypothesized and no rationale is given for the selection of one imported theoretical model over any other.

Whilst we might hope that the assembled models represent a judicious selection in a creative proliferation of workable approaches, the overall framework appears to have no guiding principles. Such unabashed eclecticism leaves health promotion in a limbo of arbitrary influences. With no theoretical basis to call its own it may be easily assimilated by more powerful rivals or dismissed as an empty subject matter wholly dependent on other disciplines.

Despite his efforts in generating core theory work, French (1990) also contends that the theoretical content of health promotion is intrinsically eclectic. He is further unhopeful about the development of any overarching health promotion theory to integrate the diverse strands of influence.

Feyerabend, however, does not sustain a pessimistic outlook with epistemological diversity. In a doctrine of proliferation he suggests scientists should proceed with an 'anything goes' philosophy. This might be best regarded as a form of brainstorming in the scientific community. Although Feyerabend's methodological and epistemological pluralism has much force in promoting a creative scientific enterprise, he ultimately neglects the objective content of science. That is, theories may in fact be successful (or not) in predicting events or giving rise to powerful technologies. The need for a solution to the demarcation problem also becomes crucial when there are rival theories vying for limited resources or where there are direct implications for social engineering (Urbach 1974). Health promotion, of course, faces exactly these circumstances.

Unlike Kuhn, Feyerabend has had little impact on social scientists, but has been influential with philosophers of science. On epistemological grounds alone, Feyerabend's position represents a logically possible extreme form of relativism, which must be taken seriously by philosophers of science. It appears that much of health promotion should also be reconsidered in the light of this epistemology.

HEALTH PROMOTION AND THE THEORY–PRACTICE GAP

Schön (1983) argues that a model of technical rationality dominates professional thinking. Practitioners can be seen to act instrumentally, applying the tools of science to solve problems. With the technical rationality of applied science, practical knowledge is entirely used as a means to an end. An assumption is made, moreover, that the ends are unambiguous and agreed upon.

Such a technical application of science in this way leads to a separation of research and practice. In turn this further polarizes the theory – practice gap, with practitioners becoming more doers than thinkers.

Since applied science is based on some scientific discipline it follows that problems are defined by the relevant scientific theory as much as the needs of practitioners. The importation of models from other disciplines in this way redefines health promotion, not as an emerging discipline growing out of the fruits of others, but as a practice ground for others. Contrary to what some advocates of the new health promotion movement think, the successful use of models imported into health promotion may not add to the discipline status of health promotion. Rather, it constitutes a victory of hegemony for the exporting discipline as it takes over further empirical ground (Laudan 1977).

Schön (1983) argues instead for the emergence of a new epistemology of practice in which practitioners reconstruct their own knowledge base from their tacit knowledge-in-action to become *reflective practitioners*. To this end he advocates incorporating into practice two sources of explicit knowledge building.

Reflection-in-action concerns knowledge which guides practice during the process of implementation. It embodies the 'tricks of the trade', or practitioner know-how.

Reflection-on-action takes a longer view and concerns the positioning of action relative to other possible courses. Both forms of reflection demand the emergence of concepts capable of encompassing practice operations. This may even necessitate the building of a new meta language to describe the basis of appropriate knowledge. Like other practitioners, health promoters have their own language, though this is largely distinct from written accounts and is only overheard in day-to-day practice or occasionally at conferences.

It is important to caution, however, against repeating the theoretical cul-de-sac encountered by educational philosophy in the attempt to deduce theory from practice. Hirst (1983) reflects that it became concerned only with explanation and neglected to produce guiding principles. De Castell (1989) adds that educational philosophy is now generally regarded as over-intellectualized and of little practical use. It led to a divide between those who had time to reflect and write, and those who could take time only to talk about their practical world. This division of labour extended yet again the distinction between theory and practice.

To articulate and codify practical knowledge, as Schön would have it, scholarly discourse must take the form of theory construction through literate practice. De Castell warns, however, that institutional factors impose severe limits upon reflections about action. Practitioners are typically given neither the time nor the encouragement to engage in theory construction.

Without some form of objectification of practice, however, it is difficult to transmit the lessons of experience efficiently. Training is almost entirely limited to role modelling. Trapped in subjective relativism each new cohort of practitioners must reinvent the subject matter (including blind alleys and mistakes) as they necessarily strive to recreate the essential experience for acquiring competence. Of greatest consequence, the growth of knowledge is severely stunted through the lack of accumulated wisdom and restricted opportunities for shared criticism.

Schön's model of the reflective practitioner cannot, moreover, be grafted on to practice in yet another exercise of technical rationality. It does, though, provide an important challenge to our view of how disciplines emerge. This is significant for training and development work amongst health promotion specialists and offers an alternative to the constricting concepts of role delineation based upon task analysis (Rawson and Grigg 1988). Just as importantly, the prospect of a new epistemology of practice shows that health promotion need not be limited by the horizons of other disciplines. There is instead the opportunity to establish core theoretical work building on the development of practice.

For health promotion theory to be regarded as progressive it must be shown to accomplish all that rival approaches claim to plus it must uncover new possibilities for improving health or at least our understanding of what constitutes health (Lakatos 1970). This will be the most difficult aspect to establish but it would also generate the most powerful indicator for continued confidence in health promotion.

CONCLUSIONS

According to Shapere (1977), in scientific practice it is rational for scientists at various stages of development of a theory to continue pursuing and fostering it even though they may be explicitly aware that it is literally false. Indeed, it may be that all young theories go through such a primitive stage and it would be nonsense to attempt refutations. Theory may be put forward initially not as true, but as some idealization or as a model or even a useful fiction. In the development of a theory it becomes pertinent to ask at any particular stage whether it purports to provide a realistic explanation or else is offered as a conceptual device. In providing an adequate account of scientific practice

Shapere also insists that we must accommodate the actual uses to which theory is put.

The same questions have to be addressed to health promotion. Even if no ready answers can be found, the asking will help better define the subject matter and create the discipline to discover the true potential of health promotion.

REFERENCES

Adams, L. (1985) 'Health education: in whose interest?', *Radical Health Promotion* Spring: 11–14.

Anderson, D. (1980) 'Blind alleys in health education', in A. Seldon (ed.) *The Litmus Papers*, London: Centre for Policy Studies.

Armistead, N. (ed.) (1974) *Reconstructing Social Psychology*, Harmondsworth: Penguin.

Bandura, A. (1977) 'Self-efficacy: towards a unifying theory of behavioural change', *Psychological Review* 84(2): 191–215.

Beattie, A. (1980) *A Structural Repertoire of the Models of Health Education*, Exeter: Health Certificate Tutors Workshop.

——(1984) 'Health education and the science teacher: an invitation to debate', *Education and Health* 2(1): 9–15.

——(1991) 'Knowledge and control in health promotion: a test case for social policy and social theory', in J. Gabe, M. Calnan, and M. Bury (eds) *The Sociology of the Health Service*, London: Routledge.

Bernstein, B. (1980) 'On the classification and framing of knowledge', in M. Young (ed.) *Knowledge and Control*, London: Collier Macmillan.

Birn, H. and Birn, B. (1985) 'Education for wellness', *Community Dental Health* 2: 1–6.

Blalock, H. M. (ed.) (1971) *Causal Models in the Social Sciences*, Chicago: Aldine Atherton.

Bowman, R. A. (1976) 'Changes in the activities, functions and roles of public health educators', *Health Education Monographs* 4(3): 226–46.

Burkitt, A. (1983) 'Models of health', in J. Clarke (ed.) *Readings in Community Medicine*, Edinburgh: Churchill Livingstone.

Burrell, G. and Morgan, G. (1985) *Sociological Paradigms and Organisational Analysis*, Aldershot: Gower.

Caplan, R. and Holland, R. (1990) 'Rethinking health education theory', *Health Education Journal* 49(1): 10–12.

de Castell, S. (1989) 'On writing of theory and practice', *Journal of the Philosophy of Education* 23(1): 39–50.

Catford, J. and Parish, R. (1989) '"Heartbeat Wales": new horizons for health promotion in the community – the philosophy and practice of Heartbeat Wales', in D. Seedhouse and A. Cribb (eds) *Changing Ideas in Health Care*, Chichester: Wiley.

Chalmers, A. F. (1976) *What is This Thing Called Science?*, Milton Keynes: Open University Press.

Collins, L. (1982) *Concepts of Health Held by Members of Four Professional Groups*, National Conference on Research and Development in Health Education with Special Reference to Youth, University of Southampton, 10 September 1982.

——(1984) 'Concepts of health education: a study of four professional groups', *Journal of Institute of Health Education* 23(3): 81–8.

Crawford, R. (1977) 'You are dangerous to your health: the ideology and politics of victim-blaming', *Journal of Health Services* 7: 663–80.

Dearden, R. F. (1972) 'Autonomy and education', in R. F. Dearden, P. H. Hurst, and R. S. Peters (eds) *Education and the Development of Reason*, London: Routledge & Kegan Paul.

Diesing, P. (1971) *Patterns of Discovery in the Social Sciences*, London: Routledge & Kegan Paul.

Dorn, N. (1983) *Alcohol, Youth and the State*, Bromley: Croom Helm.

Downie, R. S., Fyfe, C., and Tannahill, A. (1990) *Health Promotion: Models and Values*, Oxford: Oxford Medical Publications.

Draper, P. (1979) *Rethinking Community Medicine*, Unit for the Study of Health Policy, 11–15.

——(1983) 'Tackling the disease of ignorance', *Journal of College of Health* 1: 23–5.

Draper, P., Griffiths, J., Dennis, J., and Popay, J. (1979) 'Three types of health education', *British Medical Journal* 16 August: 495–8.

Dwore, R. and Matarazzo, J. (1981) 'The behavioural sciences and haelth education', *Health Education* May/June: 4–7.

Ewles, L. and Simnett, I. (1985) *Promoting Health – A practical Guide to Health Education*, Chichester: Wiley.

Feyerabend, P. (1975) *Against Method*, London: New Left Books.

Freire, P. (1972) *Pedagogy of the Oppressed*, Harmondsworth: Penguin

French, J. (1984) *A Review of Contemporary Health Education Models and their Relevance in Postgraduate Education Courses in the U.K.*, unpublished MSc dissertation, Chelsea College, University of London.

——(1990) 'Boundaries and horizons, the role of health education within health promotion', *Health Education Journal* 49(1): 7–10.

French, J. and Adams, L. (1986) 'From analysis to synthesis', *Health Education Journal* 45(2): 71–3.

Freudenberg, N. (1978) 'Shaping the future of health education from behavioural change to social action', *Health Education Monographs* 6 (4).

Galli, N. (1978) *Foundations and Principles of Health Education*, New York: Wiley

Gallie, W. B. (1956) 'Essentially contested concepts', *Proceedings of Aristotelian Society* 56: 167–98.

Gellner, E. (1974) *Legitimation of Belief*, Cambridge: Cambridge University Press.

Harré, R. (1979) *Social Being: A Theory for Social Psychology*, Oxford: Blackwell.

Hatch, S. and Kickbusch, I. (1984) *Self-help and Health in Europe*, Copenhagen: WHO.

Hirst, P. (1983) 'Educational theory', in P. Hirst (ed.) *Educational Theory and its Foundational Disciplines*, London: Routledge & Kegan Paul.

Kelvin, P. (1980) 'The search for models is a delusion', in A. J. Chapman and D. M. Jones (eds) *Models of Man*, Leicester: British Psychological Society.

Krijnen, M., Schenk, R., and Garnick, W. (eds) (1982) *Health Education – A Major in Health Science: Philosophy and Exit Level Competencies*, Limburg State University, Maastricht.

Kuhn, T. S. (1957) *The Copernican Revolution*, Boston, MA: Harvard University Press.

——(1962) *The Structure of Scientific Revolutions*, Chicago: University of Chicago Press.

——(1970) *The Structure of Scientific Revolutions*, second edition, Chicago: University of Chicago Press.

Labonte, R. and Penfold, S. (1981) 'Canadian perspectives in health promotion', *Health Education* 19: 4–7.

Lakatos, I. (1970) 'Falsification and the methodology of scientific research programmes', in I. Lakatos and A. Musgrave (eds) *Criticism and the Growth of Knowledge*, Cambridge: Cambridge University Press.

Laudan, L. (1977) *Progress and its Problems*, Berkeley, CA: University of California Press.

Manoff, R. K. (1985) *Social Marketing: New Imperatives for Public Health*, New York: Praeger.

Mills, C. Wright (1959) *The Sociological Imagination*, Oxford: Oxford University Press.

Nagel, E. (1961) *The Structure of Science*, London: Routledge & Kegan Paul.

Neutens, J. J. (1984) 'Professional competencies of the health educators', in L. Rubinson and W. F. Alles (eds) *Health Education: Foundations for the Future*, St Louis, MO: Times Mirror/Mosby.

Nutbeam, D. (1984) 'Health education in the National Health Service: the differing perspectives of community physicians and health education officers', *Health Education Journal* 43(4): 115–19.

Peters, R. S. (1977) *Education and the Education of Teachers*, London: Routledge & Kegan Paul.

Popper, K. R. (1957) *The Poverty of Historicism*, London: Routledge & Kegan Paul.

——(1959) *The Logic of Scientific Discovery*, London: Hutchinson.

——(1963) *Conjectures and Refutations*, London: Routledge & Kegan Paul.

Puska, P., Salonen, J., Nissinen, A., and Tuomilehto, J. (1983) 'Change in risk factors for coronary heart disease during ten years of community intervention programme (North Karelia Project)', *British Medical Journal* 287: 1840.

Rawson, D. and Grigg, C. (1988) *Purpose & Practice in Health Education*, London: South Bank Polytechnic/HEA.

Research Unit in Health & Behavioural Change, University of Edinburgh (1989) *Changing the Public Health*, Chichester: Wiley.

Rodmell, S. and Watts, A. (eds) (1986) *The Politics of Health Education*, London: Routledge & Kegan Paul.

Rosenberg, A. (1988) *Philosophy of Social Science*, Oxford: Clarendon Press.

Schön, D. A. (1983) *The Reflective Practitioner: How Professionals Think in Action*, New York: Basic Books.

Seedhouse, D. (1986) *Health: Foundations for Achievement*, Chichester: Wiley.

Seedhouse, D. and Cribb, A. (eds) (1989) *Changing Ideas in Health Care*, Chichester: Wiley.

Seymour, H. (1984) 'Health education versus health promotion – a practitioner's view', *Health Education Journal* 43(2&3): 37–8.

Shapere, D. (1977) 'Scientific theories and their domains', in F. Suppe (ed.) *The Structure of Scientific Theories*, Urbana: University of Illinois Press.

Slavin, H. and Chapman, V. (1985) *The Application of Models of Health Education to Health Visitor Training and Practice*, 1st International Conference of Health Education in Nursing, Health Visiting and Midwifery, Harrogate, 23 May 1985.

Smithies, J. and Adams, L., with Webster, G. and Beattie, A. (1990) *Community Participation in Health Promotion*, HEA.

Suppe, F. (ed.) (1977) *The Structure of Scientific Theories*, 2nd edition, Urbana: University of Illinois Press.

Tannahill, A. (1985) 'What is health promotion?', *Health Education Journal* 44(4): 167–8.

Taylor, V. (1990) 'Health education – a theoretical mapping', *Health Education Journal* 49(1): 13–14.

Thomas, D. (1983) *The Making of Community Work*, London: Allen & Unwin.

Thorpe, P. (1982) 'Individual or collective responsibilities for health', *Nursing* May: 8–10.

Tones, B. K. (1981) 'Health education: prevention or subversion', *Royal Society of Health Journal* 101(3): 114–17.

——(1983) 'Health education and health promotion: new directions', *Journal of Institute of Health Education* 21: 4.

——(1985) 'Health promotion – a new panacea?', *Journal of Institute of Health Education* 23: 16–21.

——(1986) 'Health education and the ideology of health promotion: a review of alternative approaches', *Health Education Research* 1(1): 3–12.

——(1990) 'Why theorize? Ideology in health education', *Health Education Journal* 49(1): 2–6.

Tones, B. K., Tilford, S., and Robinson, J. K. (1990) *Health Education: Effectiveness and Efficiency*, London: Chapman & Hall.

Urbach, P. (1974) 'Progress and degeneration in the IQ debate', *British Journal of Philosophy of Science* 25: 99–135 & 235–59.

Warr, P. B. (1980) 'An introduction to models in psychological research', in A. J. Chapman and D. M. Jones (eds) *Models of Man*, Leicester: British Psychological Society.

Whitehead, M. (1989) *Swimming Upstream: Trends and Prospects in Education and Health*, London: King's Fund Institute.

Williams, G. and Aspin, D. (1980) 'The philosophy of health education related to schools', in J. Cowley, K. David, and S. T. Williams (eds) *Health Education in Schools*, London: Harper & Row.

WHO (1984) *Health Promotion: A Discussion Document on the Concepts and Principles*, Copenhagen: WHO.

Glossary

This glossary is intended only as a guide to defining terms and readers should refer to appropriate texts for fuller explanations. All definitions are given as they relate to and are understood in health promotion theory and practice.

Acceptance variables

(Innovation-diffusion theory) These variables influence the degree or rate to which an innovation is taken up and may be divided into structural and individual variables.

Alma Ata Declaration

A declaration of the World Health Assembly at Alma Ata in the Soviet Union in 1977. The declaration committed all members of the World Health Organization to the principles of Health For All 2000 (HFA 2000).

Approach

(Theoretical debate) A term favoured by those shy of conceptual work – typically pragmatists (who focus on practicalities) and eclecticists (who mix ideas arbitrarily). Has connotations of a tentative movement.

At risk group

A group vulnerable to certain diseases or ill health because of their economic, social, or behavioural characteristics or environment. *(See Risk behaviour.)*

Audience segmentation

(*Social marketing*) The breakdown of an audience into discrete groups that show homogeneity within and heterogeneity between them. The process by which these groups are identified is arbitrary, but usually focuses on socio-economic characteristics such as social class, income, education, age, and ethnic group. Enables those marketing a message to direct it to those it is intended for, the target audience. (*See Target audience.*)

Bio-medical model

(*Sociology*) Focuses on the causes and treatment of ill health and disease in terms of biological cause and effect. This approach does not refer to the social, psychological, or economic conditions that may have influenced the health of the individual. (*See Health equity.*)

Causal attribution

(*Psychology*) The reason given for an event; to whom or to what we attribute the cause of an event. According to attribution theory, the nature of attributions made shapes future action. (*See Learned helplessness.*)

Change agent

(*Innovation-diffusion theory*) Used in relation to innovation-diffusion theory, it is defined as an individual who influences the client's innovation decision in a direction considered desirable by the change agency.

Channel gatekeepers

(*Social marketing*) Those who control the movement of messages through a communication channel, who act as intermediaries between those marketing a product or message and those it is directed at, for example, the personnel manager of a large organization. These individuals play an important part in the success or otherwise of health promotion campaigns.

Cohort

(*Epidemiology*) A component of the population born during a particular time period and identified by period of birth, so that the characteristics of this group at different points in time can be identified. More generally used to describe any group of people who are followed or traced over time. (*See Longitudinal study.*)

Conflict theory

(Sociology) The analysis of groups within society competing to serve their own conflicting interests. Fundamental to this type of analysis is the identification of inequalities between groups.

Consensus theory

(Sociology) The analysis of society as a whole, identifying the function of different groups in maintaining the equilibrium of the whole. This theory suggests that society tends to conservatism and the maintenance of the status quo.

Cost-benefit analysis

(Economics) A means of evaluating a health promotion programme by comparing costs with benefits. If benefits outweigh costs, the programme is considered efficient in cost-benefit terms. This type of analysis is limited by the problems of placing values on costs and benefits, such as the value of life or the cost of passive smoking. *(See Cost-effectiveness analysis.)*

Cost-effectiveness analysis

(Economics) Similar to cost-benefit analysis, but compares units of effectiveness to cost in order to determine the most cost-effective way of achieving programme aims. For example, if prevention of cervical cancer is the aim of a programme, a unit of effectiveness could be defined as the detection of a positive smear test, rather than the numbers of women examined. *(See Cost-benefit analysis.)*

Cross-sectional study

(Epidemiology) A study that examines the relationship between disease, ill health, and other variables of interest as they exist in a defined population at one particular point in time. This study provides a snapshot of the characteristics of the population at one point in time. *(See Longitudinal study.)*

Epidemiology

(Epidemiology) The study of the distribution and determinants of health – related states and events in populations, and the application of this study to the control of health problems.

Ethnomethodology

(Sociology) A method of enquiry in which the researcher's beliefs, attitudes, and values are accounted for in the process of research. As such, it questions the notion of scientific objectivity.

Formative research

(Social marketing) Research conducted prior to full implementation of a social marketing strategy. It may include studies of the characteristics and needs of different audience segments, pilot testing of the message or service to determine its acceptability.

Health belief model

(Psychology) A model of action describing and predicting health behaviour in terms of beliefs and perceptions about illness, the costs and benefits of action related to health, and the available cues for action. It combines links with behaviour and belief with cost-benefit analysis. *(See Cost-benefit analysis.)*

Health equity

(Sociology) Implies that ideally everyone should have a fair opportunity to attain their full health potential and that no one should be disadvantaged from achieving this potential, if it can be avoided. Equity is therefore concerned with creating equal opportunities for health and with bringing health differentials down to the lowest level possible.

Heterophily

(Communications theory) The degree to which pairs of individuals who interact are different with regard to certain attributes. *(See Homophily.)*

Homophily

(Communications theory) Used in innovation-diffusion theory in relation to the characteristics of the change agent and his or her client group. When they share certain characteristics they are said to be homophilous and it is argued that under these conditions more effective communication occurs.

Iatrogenesis

The occurrence of illness as a result of earlier treatment by a doctor, or other health care worker, for a previous illness.

Innovation

An idea, object, or practice perceived as new by the individual to whom the innovation is targeted. *(See Innovation-diffusion theory.)*

Innovation-diffusion theory

(Communications theory) A theory in which the process by which an innovation spreads through society is identified. Typically this follows an 'S' curve, slowly at first, then more rapidly, and finally slowing down again. It is useful to health promotion as different social groups play different roles in the uptake of an innovation, and their identification and allegiance can play an important role in the eventual success of a programme. *(See Innovation, Change agent, Pro-innovation bias, Acceptance variables.)*

Intermittent reinforcement

(Psychology) An unpredictable schedule of reinforcement (rewards) which may exert a powerful effect on behaviour. For example, when the discomfort and unpleasant consequences of binge drinking are interspersed with occasional euphoric and enjoyable experiences, drinking may be perceived as enjoyable and repeated.

Lay beliefs

(Sociology) Non-professional interpretations of the causes and treatment of ill health and disease and the reasons for susceptibility. They are frequently inconsistent, differing with the level of explanation required (contrasts with bio-medical model).

Learned helplessness

(Psychology) A learnt response to unpleasant experiences beyond individual control. It is characterized by apathy and inability to avoid further unpleasant experiences. Generalization to other situations may occur and the behaviour may persist over time. This depends on the causal attribution made for the experience. *(See Causal attribution.)*

Longitudinal study

(Epidemiology) Sometimes called a cohort study. A study in which the same group of people are observed at different points in time.

Marketing mix

(Social marketing) The relative emphasis placed on the product, place, promotion, and price in a given marketing strategy. The different importance given to these factors is determined by the characteristics of the target audience. An effective marketing mix optimizes the communication of the message, service, or product being marketed.

Model

(Theoretical debate) A misused word – sometimes interchanged with theory, perspective, approach, and position. Refers to temporary conceptual constructions used to assist our thinking, more primitive than theories but perhaps embodying propositions, hypotheses, etc.

Morbidity

(Epidemiology) Any departure from a state of health or well-being, whether physiological or psychological. It can be measured by the numbers in a population who are ill, the periods of illness these people experienced, and the types of illness that these people suffered.

Multivariate analysis

(Epidemiology) A set of techniques used when the variation in several variables has to be measured at the same time. In statistics it is any analytical method that allows the simultaneous study of two or more dependent variables.

Naturalism

(Sociology) A position which supports the idea that people are intrinsically good and, if set free from the trappings and constraints of society, healthy development will automatically emerge. This position is usually connected with Rousseau.

Opinion leaders

(Communication theory) A social group playing a central role in the uptake of innovations. They are characteristically respected, with good communication systems their behaviour has an impact on their community, and they are identifiable as the key movers in the early uptake of new ideas, actions, and technology. *(See Innovation-diffusion theory.)*

Opportunity cost

(Economics) The cost of production judged by what has been forgone by not using resources in another way. In health promotion the cost could be a service, a new behaviour, or a product. For example, the opportunity cost of taking exercise would include the loss of benefits from using the time for other activities.

Paradigm

(Theory, philosophy) A wider concept than theory. It constitutes the agreed upon way of looking at and interpreting the world, or a particular field of study, and predicts the course of further investigation and study. A theoretical paradigm refers to the context within which a theory exists; two rival theories may share the same paradigm. For example, psychoanalysis and transactional analysis are both part of the psychodynamic paradigm, as they share fundamental similarities in their understanding of emotional life and how emotional problems may be cured.

Paradigm shift

(Theory, philosophy) Refers to the way in which one paradigm is replaced by another (Kuhn 1970). According to Kuhn, there are three stages in this process of scientific development: a pre-paradigm stage when several theories compete for dominance, then a period of normal science when a single paradigm has gained wide acceptance and provides structure for the field. This is followed by a period of crisis, when the accepted paradigm is replaced by another. This is called the paradigm shift; it is a revolution in thinking and in knowledge.

Perspective

(Theoretical debate) A term favoured by theorists to describe the unique qualities of their work. Best thought of as describing their epistemological basis (core assumptions about how their theoretical knowledge is generated).

Position

(Theoretical debate) A term favoured by activists (who see theorizing as wasteful effort). Usually associated with a 'defence' of a position or developing a 'sound' position (meaning ideologically acceptable).

Process tracking

(Social marketing) Systematic measurement of effectiveness, in reaching and delivering a message to the target audience of a social marketing programme. It provides a means of assessing whether or not the aims and objectives of the programme are being met and the impact of the programme as a whole. *(See Target audience.)*

Pro-innovation bias

(Communications theory) The assumption by those researching or promoting an innovation that it is beneficial before it has been proven to be so. This usually occurs when alternatives have not been examined and can be remedied by the use of control groups and different experimental conditions for testing the innovation. Fosters a victim-blaming view if the innovation is not adopted. *(See Victim blaming.)*

Reference population

(Epidemiology) Equivalent to a control group (a group who have not been exposed to the conditions manipulated for study) or comparison group in studies observing populations.

Risk behaviour

Specific forms of behaviour known to be associated with increased susceptibility to certain diseases or ill health. In health promotion, changes to risk behaviour are a major goal in disease prevention. *(See At risk group.)*

Saliency

(Communication theory) In the context of innovation adoption, the more salient or obvious the advantage, adoptability, or accessibility of an innovation, then the more likely it is that the innovation will be taken up. *(See Innovation-diffusion theory.)*

Self-regulation theory

(Psychology) Suggests the regulation of health-threatening behaviour occurs by active recall of the long-term consequences of the behaviour. This theory may be used in developing training programmes, such as alcohol counselling services, as it enables individuals to self-regulate their own health behaviour.

Sensitivity analysis

(Economics) Used to determine the sensitivity of cost-benefit analysis to changes in the assumptions on which it is based. It identifies those conditions around which most uncertainty exists, then alters their values. The analysis gives an indication of the degree of confidence one can have in the results of the cost-benefit analysis. *(See Cost-benefit analysis.)*

Social stratification

(Sociology) Persistent divisions identified in society that are resistant to change and are usually characterized by socio-economic factors, such as level of skill in employment, income, and education. The stratification of society may be said to be a structural characteristic as it is resistant to change.

Stages of change model

(Psychology) Identifies five major stages in effecting behavioural change: pre-contemplation, contemplation, ready for action, action, and maintenance. The model is dynamic and it is possible to move back and forth between stages. Different processes are involved at different stages, enabling health promoters to provide appropriate support. For example, awareness raising at the pre-contemplation stage, coping skills for those ready for action, and positive reinforcement and continued encouragement for those maintaining a behavioural change.

Statistical lives

(Economics) A term used to describe lives that do not exist, but are used in forecasting the future for statistical purposes, for example, the probable number of lives lost in road accidents next year or the number of children whose lives could be saved through screening pregnant women for certain diseases.

Structuralism

(Sociology) An examination of the constraints placed on behaviour and social action by the environment in which the action occurs. Its areas of concern are, for example, local and national government, laws, taxation, and the planning of the built environment.

Target audience

(Social marketing) The group to whom a marketing programme is being directed. It is separated from the audience as a whole by identifying it by key characteristics, for example, age, sex, and social class.

Taxonomies

(Theoretical debate) Categorical classifications of elements into different species or groups.

Theories

(Theoretical debate) Organized or integrated sets of propositions, better thought of as a 'theoretical system' in contrast to the above terms. Synonymous with explanatory system. Retains etymology of 'composition' and 'speculation' (same origin as spectator, spectacle, etc., meaning viewpoint or perspective).

Typologies

(Theoretical debate) Dimensional classification with a continuously graded array of elements. Typological labels usually given to the extremes or polarities.

Vicarious learning

(Psychology) Learning by observing others without direct experience. For example, smoking in children may be learnt vicariously as it is portrayed as an enjoyable/desirable activity by the media or by contemporaries at school.

Victim blaming

Health-promoting activities based on the belief that problems with health are the responsibility of the individual and not the social or economic environment in which the individual finds him or herself. *(See Pro-innovation bias.)*

Name index

Abramson, L.Y. 26
Adams, L. 202, 207, 209, 211, 215, 216
Aggleton, P. 16, 29, 61, 73, 100
Ajzen, I. 24
Altman, D.G. 124
Anderson, J. 72
Andreasen, A.R. 160–1, 168
Armstrong, D. 8, 46, 52
Ashton, J. 51, 61, 73, 134
Aspey, D. 79
Atkin, C.K. 162, 165

Bandura, A. 16, 24, 76, 167, 218
Barker, D.J.P. 86, 93
Basaglia, F.O. 9
Beattie, A. 2, 129, 207, 208, 211, 212
Becker, M.H. 27, 77
Beeles, C. 72
Bernstein, B. 16, 211
Birn, H. and Birn, B. 213
Black Committee 50–1
Blalock, H.M. 209
Blaxter, M. 47, 48, 51
Bloom, P.N. 165, 179
Blum, H.L. 135
Brown, L.A. 185
Bunton, R. 135, 141
Burkitt, A. 213

Canfield, J. 78
Catford, J. 39, 207, 217, 218
Central Council for Health Education
    10, 11
Chadwick, E. 10
Chalmers, A.F. 204
Chapman, V. 216
Charles, N. 58

Cohen, D.R. 113, 118, 122, 123
Collins, L. 207
Coopersmith, B. 79
Cornwell, J. 47, 49, 51
Cullis, J.G. 116
Cummings, S.R. 125

Davey-Smith, G. 51
Dawber, T.R. 92
de Castell, S. 219–20
Dept. of Health and Social Security
    (DHSS) 50, 144, 145
DiClemente, C.C. 27–8
Diesing, P. 210
Doll, R. 91, 92, 122
Doremus Porter Novelli 162
Dorn, N. 54, 71, 73, 207
Downie, R.S. 95, 100, 207, 210, 213,
    214, 217
Durkheim, E. 44

Ewles, L. 145, 210–11, 217

Farmer, R.D.T. 88
Farquhar, J.W. 170
Feyerabend, P. 217–18
Fine, S.H. 153, 157, 158, 159, 163
Fishbein, M. 16, 24
Flora, J.A. 153, 154–5, 156, 162, 164,
    169, 170, 173
Foucault, M. 14, 45, 47
Freire, P. 68, 69, 215
French, J. 207, 208, 209, 211, 216, 218
Freudenberg, N. 215

Galdston, I. 102
Gellner, E. 205

Subject index